Cover design by Judy McHenry

W0234996

First published in 2004 by Lawrence Erlbaum Associates Inc.

Published in 2015 by Routledge
605 Third Avenue, New York, NY 10017
4 Park Square, Milton Park, Abingdon Oxon OX14 4RN

Routledge is an imprint of the Taylor & Francis Group, an informa business.

ISBN: 9781138424876 (hbk)
ISBN: 9780805895308 (pbk)

HUMAN PERFORMANCE
Volume 17, Number 3, 2004

SPECIAL ISSUE: Personality and the Prediction of
Job Performance: More Than the Big Five
Walter C. Borman, *Guest Editor*

HUMAN PERFORMANCE, *17*(3), 267–269

Introduction to the Special Issue. Personality and the Prediction of Job Performance: More Than the Big Five

Walter C. Borman

Associate Editor, Human Performance
PDRI and University of South Florida

Personality in industrial/organizational (I/O) psychology was dealt a near death blow in 1965 by the Guion and Gottier (1965) critique of the use of personality inventories in personnel selection. Reaction to the article by the I/O community was perhaps overdone, but it resulted in a considerable reduction in personality-related research within the personnel selection context. In 1991, however, all that changed. Barrick and Mount (1991) and Tett, Jackson, and Rothstein (1991) both reviewed relations between personality at the Big Five level (i.e., Extraversion, Agreeableness, Conscientiousness, Emotional stability, and Openness to experience) and job performance. These reviews were more positive about the validity of personality for predicting performance and helped create (especially Barrick & Mount, 1991) a more favorable climate for I/O research focused on personality.

Further, there is little doubt that I/O psychology has embraced the Big Five as an organizing framework for personality in personnel selection. At one level, this is good, because if the Big Five is used consistently in personnel selection research, we obtain cumulative evidence regarding personality–performance links, more so than if different investigators employ different personality constructs. However, rigid adherence to the Big Five model is probably not wise for our field. For example, there is some evidence that narrower personality constructs will correlate higher with relatively specific criteria (e.g., Crant, 1995; Hogan & Roberts, 1996; Schneider & Hough, 1995) and this is highly desirable for the science of personnel selection (Borman, Hanson, & Hedge, 1997). There is also evidence that broader constructs may be better in some contexts, especially when the target criteria are very broad (Ones & Viswesvaran, 1996). Integrity is a good example. Meta-analysis shows substantial validity for this composite of Conscientiousness,

Emotional Stability, and Agreeableness against overall job performance criteria (Ones, Viswesvaran, & Schmidt, 1993).

The three primary articles in this special issue explore personality measurement in both directions; that is, more narrow and specific and more broad and heterogeneous. First, Larry James reviews his research program on *conditional reasoning*, with a focus on the construct of aggression. This is the second construct measured by James and colleagues using the conditional reasoning paradigm. James, McIntyre, Glisson, Bowler, and Mitchell present data on a series of studies that show quite high relations, consistently higher than the Big Five has provided, between Aggression and a variety of criteria conceptually associated with this construct. Also presented are data that suggest good construct validity for the measure. Finally, there is reason to believe that the conditional reasoning approach to personality measurement may reduce problems with slanting of responses or faking in a selection setting.

David Chan moves even farther away from the Big Five by exploring a construct he calls *tolerance for contradiction*. It is defined as a mode of thinking that accepts and even thrives on apparent contradictory information. Chan demonstrates that although the construct does not itself correlate with job performance, it successfully moderates the relation between situation judgment tests and job performance. Specifically, tolerance for contradiction correlates positively with performance when situational judgment ability is high and negatively with performance when situational judgment ability is low. Accordingly, this construct can be either adaptive or maladaptive, depending on one's level of situational judgment ability.

Tim Judge and his colleagues have been studying a construct they refer to as *core self-evaluation* (CSE; e.g., Judge & Bono, 2001). Judge, Van Vianen, and De Pater combine measures of four traits: locus of control, self-esteem, generalized self-efficacy, and emotional stability to form this "mega-construct." Importantly, as part of their research program, Judge et al. seek to understand why personality relates to job performance and job satisfaction. For example, they have shown that high CSE contributes to job satisfaction because those high on CSE generally obtain more complex and challenging jobs. Also, with the complexity of the job held constant, high CSE workers perceive their jobs as more challenging and interesting, thus contributing to job satisfaction.

In the final article in this issue, Neal Schmitt provides a provocative and insightful critique and commentary of the three primary articles. In his review, Schmitt notes some important points of criticism, but is primarily positive and laudatory of these research programs. One of his main observations on personality research in the personnel selection arena is that Big Five job performance relations are actually quite low, with the highest correlations (between conscientiousness and job performance) in the mid .20s, even with corrections applied. Thus, there does seem to be a need to move beyond the Big Five. Overall, Schmitt views favorably the three research programs described in this issue as promising adjuncts to existing personality measures.

In closing, I thank our authors for preparing these fine articles. The three substantive articles are important contributions to the personality–job performance literature and the commentary provides an insightful perspective on the topic. Thanks also to an anonymous reviewer who provided excellent reviews of all three articles and to Jim Farr, who also provided constructive feedback on all of the articles.

REFERENCES

Barrick, M. R., & Mount, M. K. (1991). The Big Five personality dimensions and job performance: A meta-analysis. *Personnel Psychology, 44,* 1–26.

Borman, W. C., Hanson, M. A., & Hedge, J. W. (1997). Personnel selection. In J. T. Spence, J. M. Darley, & D. J. Foss (Eds.), *Annual review of psychology* (Vol. 48, pp. 299–337). Palo Alto, CA: Annual Review.

Crant, J. M. (1995). The proactive personality scale and objective job performance among real estate agents. *Journal of Applied Psychology, 80,* 532–537.

Guion, R. M., & Gottier, R. F. (1965). Validity of personality measures in personnel selection. *Personnel Psychology, 18,* 135–164.

Hogan, J., & Roberts, B (1996). Issues and non-issues in the fidelity–bandwidth trade-off. *Journal of Organisational Behaviour, 17,* 627–637

Judge, T. A., & Bono, J. E. (2001). A rose by any other name: Are neuroticism, self-esteem, locus of control, and generalized self-efficacy indicators of a common construct? In B. W. Roberts & R. T. Hogan (Eds.), *Personality psychology in the workplace* (pp. 93–118). Washington, DC: American Psychological Association.

Ones, D. S., & Viswesvaran, C. (1996). Bandwidth–fidelity in personality measurement for personnel selection. *Journal of Organisational Behaviour 17,* 609–626

Ones, D. S., Viswesvaran, C., & Schmidt, F. L. (1993). Comprehensive meta-analysis of integrity test validities: Findings and implications for personnel selection and theories of job performance. *Journal of Applied Psychology (Monograph), 78,* 679–703.

Schneider, R., & Hough L. (1995). Personality and industrial/organizational psychology. In C. Cooper & I. Robertson (Eds.), *International review of industrial and organizational psychology,* (pp. 75–129). Chichester, England: Wiley.

Tett, R., Jackson, D., & Rothstein, M. (1991). Personality measures as predictors of job performance: A meta-analytic review. *Personnel Psychology, 44,* 703–742.

HUMAN PERFORMANCE, *17*(3), 271–295

The Conditional Reasoning Measurement System for Aggression: An Overview

Lawrence R. James, Michael D. McIntyre, Charles A. Glisson, and Jennifer L. Bowler

Industrial–Organizational Psychology Program
University of Tennessee

Terence R. Mitchell

Department of Management
University of Washington

The Conditional Reasoning Measurement System is described. This procedure focuses on how people solve what on the surface appear to be inductive reasoning problems. The true intent of the problems is to determine if solutions based on implicit biases are logically attractive to a respondent. In this article, we focus on the types of implicit biases that underlie aggressive individuals' attempts to justify aggressive behavior. People who consistently select solutions based on these types of biases are scored as being potentially aggressive because they are cognitively prepared to rationalize aggression. Scores on the Conditional Reasoning Test for Aggression (CRT-A) have been shown to have acceptable psychometric properties and an average, uncorrected validity of .44 against behavorial criteria (in 10 studies).

Many waking hours are spent thinking inductively. What is the best investment strategy for retirement in the present financial climate? Is war with Middle Eastern countries inevitable and what will be the outcomes of war? Which is more conducive to education, public schools or private schools? What will happen if the price of gas increases to two or more dollars a gallon? For each problem, one determines which conclusion, or perhaps conclusions, follows reasonably from a set of pre-

Requests for reprints should be sent to Lawrence R. James, School of Psychology and College of Management, Georgia Institute of Technology, Atlanta, GA 30332. E-mail: ljames@utk.edu

mises (i.e., evidence, assumptions, advocacies, or arguments). Specifically, one assesses which evidence is credible, which assumptions are tenable, which arguments are valid, and, ultimately, which conclusion(s) is most likely to be true. This is inductive reasoning, although it focuses less on formal problem solving than on the deliberations that people use everyday to attempt to make sense of their environments and to decide on reasonable ways to adapt to those environments (Galotti, 1989; Kuhn, 1991; Wagner & Sternberg, 1985, 1986).

A significant portion of everyday reasoning attempts to determine what reasonable people would do when faced with frustrating or threatening circumstances. For example, what would reasonable people do upon learning that their jobs are about to be downsized? How would reasonable people react to being kept awake at night by the barking of a neighbor's dog? What is a reasonable response to being hit from behind while sitting in a car at a stoplight? What is a reasonable amount of time to wait in an examining room for a physician to appear?

People will differ in what they consider reasonable responses in each of these situations. However, the array of individual conclusions will, for normal people, be bounded by the cultural norms (i.e., standards) and cultural values (i.e., ideologies and rationales that support the norms) that define prosocial or socially adaptive behavior in our society (James & Mazerolle, 2002; Wright & Mischel, 1987). Basically, the inferences prosocial people make about reasonable behavior are shaped by having been socialized into a culture, which is to say having internalized the culture's norms, ideologies, and rationales. Inferences consistent with cultural norms, ideologies, and rationales are taken to be reasonable, sound, and sensible (Kuhn, 1991).

JUSTIFICATION OF AGGRESSIVE BEHAVIOR

With this cognitive mindset, prosocial individuals typically find it difficult to understand why people engage in aggressive, antisocial behavior. Why would some people shoot their coworkers or neighbors (or neighbor's dog)? Why would some people steal major items from their company? Why would some students vandalize their own schools? Why do some people continuously engage in spreading malicious gossip? Why do some people try to control and dominate others? Why are some people habitually absent or tardy? How do some people justify deliberately inferior performance?

Nothing in the cognitive repertoire used by prosocial people to determine the bounds of reasonable behavior prepares them to answer these questions. All they can say is that each of the behaviors is dysfunctional and socially deviant according to the standards of their culture, which engenders judgments that the people who are responsible for the behaviors must be irrational or foolish. Prosocial people would, therefore, be even more mystified to learn that the individuals who perpetrate aggressive behaviors often think of their actions as reasonable (see Anderson, 1994; Baron & Richardson, 1994; Baumeister, Smart, & Boden, 1996; Crick & Dodge, 1994; Felson & Tedeschi, 1993; Huesmann, 1988; James, 1998; Toch, 1993).

For example, people who attack their coworkers often regard their violence as justifiable acts of retaliation for having been persecuted and victimized by their peers. The chain of logic that leads to this justification typically begins with future aggressors framing interactions with coworkers as contests to establish dominance versus submissiveness (Gay, 1993; James & Mazerolle, 2002; Tedeschi & Nesler, 1993). Coworkers are categorized as (a) strong, powerful, and threatening; or (b) weak, compliant, and submissive. The latter coworkers are regarded as easily intimidated, whereas the threatening coworkers are thought of as potential intimidators and persecutors. Aggressive people reason that confronting potential intimidators is more reasonable than cooperating with them because cooperation shows weakness and invites being persecuted and bullied (Anderson, 1994; Baron & Richardson, 1994; Crick & Dodge, 1994). Confrontation, on the other hand, is thought to demonstrate power, potency, and forcefulness, which function to discourage potential persecutors from attempting to victimize the aggressive individuals.

To justify confrontation, aggressive people seek out evidence of hostile intent on the part of coworkers. They notice that coworkers often offer assistance. However, they decipher that the true intent of these offers is for coworkers to gain access to their work so that they can sabotage it. If sabotage is not possible, then by assisting, the coworkers can take all or most of the credit for the aggressive individuals' work. Further evidence that they—the aggressive individuals—are victims of exploitation, injustice, and oppression is given by coworkers' attempts to undermine their credibility with supervisors by blaming them whenever something goes wrong. Being unaware of the persecution by coworkers, the supervisors critique the aggressive individuals' work, which both angers them for its injustice and makes them feel inadequate. Injustice and inadequacy are potent fuels for anger and aggression.

The thinking of aggressive people focuses progressively on how to seek retribution and get even for the wounded pride, persecution, and disrespect that they believe they have suffered at the hands of coworkers. Some form of aggression is judged to be reasonable and justified because it offers a means to restore respect and to exact restitution for these perceived wrongs (cf. Bradbury & Fincham, 1990; Dodge, 1986; Laursen & Collins, 1994; Nisbett, 1993). Acts of retribution can take many forms, including verbal aggression (e.g., threats, character assassination, intimidation, spreading of malicious gossip), physical aggression (e.g., shoving, fighting, attacks with weapons), or passive aggression (e.g., intentional nonattendance at team meetings, deliberate failure to return messages).

The reasoning of our illustrative aggressive individuals differs considerably from the reasoning that would be expected by prosocial individuals. Where aggressive individuals frame coworkers as either submissive or potential persecutors, prosocial individuals see potential colleagues or even friends. Where aggressive individuals think that confrontation is logically preferable to cooperation, prosocial people would conclude that confrontation is unreasonable because it serves as a catalyst for overt and continued conflict. Cooperation, reconciliation, and compromise would be deemed more rational choices because they defuse anger and promote long-term peace. Finally, where aggressive individuals see hostile intent and the desire to victimize them, prosocial individuals see more benign intent underlying the actions of coworkers. Thus, prosocial people are much less likely than aggressive people to see injustices, feel anger, or experience urges to aggress.

Basically, aggressive individuals differ from prosocial individuals in terms of the adjectives they use to frame coworkers, the behaviors of their coworkers they select as being relevant indicators of their coworkers' intentions, the assumptions they make about why coworkers behave as they do, and the arguments for and against aggression they judge to be valid. These differences highlight the fact that the framing and reasoning of aggressive individuals is designed to justify aggression; that is, its intent is to enhance the rational appeal of engaging in behavior that harms others. Aggressive people are generally unaware of this intent. As noted earlier, they believe their reasoning is rational. They can engage in this self-deception because the biasing of their reasoning toward rationalizing aggression occurs below the surface of their consciousness. Specifically, the reasoning of aggressive people is implicitly (unconsciously) shaped by biases whose function is to enhance the rational appeal of aggression. James (1998; James & Mazerolle, 2002) proposed the term *justification mechanisms* (JMs) to identify these implicit biases.

JUSTIFICATION MECHANISMS

We have identified six JMs as being instrumental in rationalizing the expression of aggression. These six JMs are summarized in Table 1. Each of these JMs allows aggressive people to foster the unrealistic self-concept that they can behave aggressively and remain moral, socially adaptive, and capable of self-control. Rationalizing aggression is accordingly an act of self-deception that (a) is intended to conceal from awareness the true but unacceptable cause of aggression, namely a strong desire to inflict harm, whereas (b) sparing aggressive individuals the anxiety and guilt of self-perceptions that they are hostile, malicious, or malevolent (see James & Mazerolle, 2002). Basically, each JM is a specific facet of the defense mechanism of rationalization that allows aggressive people to enhance the rational appeal of behaviors that express their desire to inflict harm on others (see James, 1998).

TABLE 1
Justification Mechanisms Used to Develop Conditional Reasoning
Measurement System for Aggression

1. Hostile attribution bias: Tendency to see malevolent intent in actions of others. Even benign or friendly acts may be seen as having hidden, hostile agendas designed intentionally to inflict harm. An especially virulent form of this bias occurs when benign or positive acts are attributed to selfish concerns and negative incentives (e.g., a helpful suggestion by a supervisor is interpreted by an aggressive subordinate as an intentional attempt to demean his or her work).

2. Derogation of target bias: An attempt to make the target more deserving of aggression. For example, a number of negative characteristics may be ascribed to the target (e.g., corrupt, dishonest, evil, immoral, underhanded, unethical, untrustworthy). Or, the positive traits of the target may be ignored, undervalued, or depreciated.

3. Retribution bias: Tendency to confer logical priority to reparation or retaliation over reconciliation. Reflected in implicit beliefs that aggression is warranted to restore respect or exact restitution for a perceived wrong. Bias is also indicated by whether a person would rather retaliate than forgive, be vindicated as opposed to cooperate, and obtain revenge rather than maintain a relationship. This bias underlies classic rationalizations for aggression based on wounded pride, challenged self-esteem, and disrespect.

4. Victimization by powerful others bias: Tendency to frame self as a victim and to see self as being exploited and taken advantage of by the powerful (e.g., government agencies). Sets the stage for arguing that aggression is acting out against injustice, correcting an inequity, redressing wrongs, or striking out against oppression.

5. Potency bias: Tendency to frame and reason using the contrast of strength versus weakness. For example, people with a strong potency bias tend to frame others on a continuum ranging from (a) strong, assertive, powerful, daring, fearless, or brave to (b) weak, impotent, submissive, timid, sheepish, compliant, conforming, or cowardly. This bias is used to justify aggression via arguments such as (a) aggression (e.g., confrontations with teachers, fights with coworkers), which results in being perceived as brave or as a leader by others; and (b) weakness/submissiveness, which invites aggression because it shows that one is willing to submit.

6. Social discounting bias: Tendency to call on socially unorthodox and frequently antisocial beliefs to interpret and analyze social events and relationships. Disdainful of traditional ideals and conventional beliefs. Insensitive, unempathetic, unfettered by social customs. Directly cynical or critical, with few subliminal channels for routing antisocial framing and analyses.

Several of the JMs in Table 1 feature prominently in the reasoning of our illustrative aggressive individuals. The Potency Bias, for example, implicitly directs conscious framing and reasoning toward thinking of interactions with others as contests to establish dominance versus submissiveness. One result is, as we have seen, a tendency to view coworkers as weak or strong, the latter being potential persecutors. The Potency Bias is also instrumental in promoting reasoning that confrontation is more reasonable than cooperation. The Hostile Attribution Bias works below the surface of consciousness to promote hostile intent and malevolent purpose as the causes for coworkers' behaviors. This bias is often responsible for justifications of aggression based on self-defense. As a final example, the Retribution Bias tacitly advances seeking retaliation as a more reasonable reaction to a perceived wrong than seeking reconciliation or attempting to maintain a working relationship. Aggression is thought to be justified because it is intended to restore respect and assuage wounded pride.

How is it possible to determine whether JMs are instrumental in shaping a person's reasoning and, therefore, predisposing him or her to behave aggressively? The major stumbling block to developing a system of measurement for JMs is that the biases in Table 1 operate unconsciously. By virtue of being implicit and thus hidden from introspection, JMs cannot be assessed by the popular method of self-report (Nisbett & Wilson, 1977; Schwarz, 1999; Winter, John, Stewart, Klohnen, & Duncan, 1998). People cannot describe or report on psychological mechanisms that operate outside of their consciousness. (Nor can they control or manipulate or lie about that which they are unaware.)

One approach to measuring JMs would be to study a person's reasoning over time and across different situations to determine if recurrent themes such as the Hostile Attribution Bias are evident. Data on reasoning could be obtained via repeated interviews or written reports. This approach is cumbersome, time-consuming, and inefficient, and would be useful primarily in clinical settings.

CONDITIONAL REASONING

A more efficient approach is to use a new psychological measurement system designed specifically to determine whether JMs are instrumental in shaping a person's reasoning. This system was proposed recently by James (1998). It assesses whether reasoning known to be produced by JMs for aggression is judged by respondents to be logical or illogical (see also James & McIntyre, 2000; James & Mazerolle, 2002; James & Rentsch, in press). This assessment is based on a new type of inductive reasoning problem. These problems are analogous to traditional inductive reasoning tasks in that respondents are asked to determine which general conclusion follows most reasonably from a set of premises (e.g., Sternberg, 1984).

A problem designed for entry-level jobs is as follows:

The old saying, "an eye for an eye," means that if someone hurts you, then you should hurt that person back. If you are hit, then you should hit back. If someone burns your house, then you should burn that person's house.

Which of the following is the biggest problem with the "eye for an eye" plan?

(a) It tells people to "turn the other cheek."
(b) It offers no way to settle a conflict in a friendly manner.
(c) It can only be used at certain times of the year.
(d) People have to wait until they are attacked before they can strike.

Respondents believe that their critical intellectual skills guide their attempts to identify a logically correct conclusion to this problem. But the true demands of this inductive reasoning task are only partially intellectual (and this demand is quite modest). The bulk of the demand appears intellectual but in fact is produced by a tacit requirement to judge whether reasoning based on a JM is more or less reasonable than reasoning based on more temperate, prosocial ideologies and rationales.

That is to say, respondents see an inductive reasoning problem that they believe to be comprised by objectively true and false conclusions. This problem is actually comprised by a conclusion drawn from JMs and a conclusion drawn from the prosocial counterparts to JMs (plus two illogical conclusions). When respondents engage in inductive reasoning to identify which conclusion is rational and which are irrational (or less rational), they think that their reasoning is determined by their inductive reasoning skills. In truth, their reasoning is guided by their respective implicit assumptions about what constitutes rational behavior. Thus, in a manner analogous to everyday reasoning about the rationality of aggression, what is judged to be the most reasonable answer to each problem is conditional on whether or not underlying biases (i.e., JMs) implicitly shape reasoning.

Basically, there are two possible solutions to each problem. One of these solutions offers an inference whose logical credibility is *conditional on reasoning being shaped by a JM or set of JMs.* Alternative (d) illustrates this case. The reasoning offered in this solution appears logically plausible to someone whose reasoning is implicitly shaped by the Retribution Bias and the Victimization (by Powerful Others) Bias. In other words, this alternative is logically attractive to aggressive individuals because it (a) tacitly promotes retribution as being logically preferable to reconciliation and (b) is grounded in the unstated assumption that the powerful will inflict harm on the less powerful unless the less powerful strike first. Selection of Alternative (d) as the most logically persuasive of the conclusions offered provides indirect evidence that the Retribution Bias and Victimization Bias are implicitly instrumental in shaping the reasoning of a respondent.

We hasten to note that some respondents may select Alternative (d) for reasons that differ from those cited earlier. We do not, therefore, place undue weight on the responses to a single problem. What is important for measurement is whether a respondent consistently selects reasoning based on JMs across a set of problems that vary in terms of inductive argument and subject matter.

It is expected that nonaggressive respondents will reject Alternative (d) as extreme and unnecessarily provocative even though it appears to follow logically from the premises. Alternative (b) is targeted to appeal to nonaggressive individuals' desire for a more prosocial alternative to counterbalance the antagonistic and provocative tenor of Alternative (d). This inference follows logically from the premises but lacks the cynicism and enmity of Alternative (d). It offers an option whose logical credibility is *conditional on reasoning being shaped by prosocial ideologies and rationales.* Selection of Alternative (b) provides indirect evidence that the Retribution Bias and Victimization Bias are not implicitly instrumental in shaping reasoning.

To enhance the face validity of the task, and to protect the indirect nature of measurement, Alternatives (a) and (c) were added to the problem. These conclusions are meant to be clearly illogical and rejected by respondents (which is usually the case). In regard to possible solutions to the problem, Alternative (d) is referred to as the "AG" alternative because it is designed to appeal to aggressive individuals. Alternative (b) is targeted for nonaggressive individuals and is referred to as the "NA" alternative.

Problems such as the one illustrated earlier are referred to as *conditional reasoning problems* because how each is solved is dependent on whether (or to what degree) JMs for aggression are instrumental in shaping reasoning. This psychometric approach is referred to as the *Conditional Reasoning Measurement System* (James, 1998).

Our objective over the last 10 or so years has been to develop a system to measure the extent to which JMs influence a person's reasoning. James (1998) suggested that if we could measure whether reasoning is implicitly influenced by the JMs that serve a strong desire or motive to aggress, then we could use the measurements to make inferences about the relative strength of the underlying need to hurt or harm others. This in turn would afford us the opportunity to make valid diagnoses of personality dispositions, especially motive-based dispositions that people often reject, deny, or are unaware of (i.e., are implicit), such as aggressiveness. Valid measurement could also enhance our understanding of the cognitive underpinnings of personality, particularly implicit functions that are not subject to introspection. Finally, and perhaps most important, valid assessment of whether a person is cognitively prepared to justify aggression by having JMs in place substantially increases our ability to predict whether that person is likely to engage in aggression in the future.

Conditional Reasoning Test for Aggression (CRT–A)

The Conditional Reasoning Test for Aggression (CRT–A) is composed of 22 conditional reasoning (CR) problems (James & McIntyre, 2000). The 22 CR problems in the CRT–A evolved over a series of developmental studies, including 10 empirical validation studies. Each CR problem was based on one or more of the six JMs. To be considered for retention, a CR problem had to significantly predict behavioral indicators of aggression, preferably in more than one sample.

Several methods were examined for scoring the 22 CR problems. These alternatives provided highly correlated scores and essentially equal correlations with external variables. However, the method described later produced the most interpretable factor structure.

Respondents are given a "+1" for every AG alternative they select (i.e., alternatives based on JMs), a "0" for every logically incorrect alternative they select (an infrequent event), and a "−1" for every NA alternative they select (i.e., alternatives based on prosocial counterparts to JMs). These scores are summed to furnish a composite score on the Conditional Reasoning–Aggression Scale (CR–A). A high score on the CR–A scale indicates that JMs for aggression are instrumental in guiding and shaping a respondent's reasoning. A proclivity to reason in ways that justify aggression suggests that the respondent is implicitly prepared and willing to engage in some form of aggressive behavior in the future (James, 1998; James & Mazerolle, 2002; James & McIntyre, 2000).

A low score on the CR–A scale indicates that JMs are not instrumental in guiding and shaping a respondent's reasoning. In contrast to those with high scores, a weak or nonexistent proclivity to reason in ways that tacitly justify aggression suggests that the respondent is not implicitly prepared and willing to engage in aggressive behavior.

Scores ranging between the weak and strong poles on the CR–A scale indicate selection of a few but not a large number of AG alternatives (compared to other respondents). JMs appear to be only sporadically instrumental in shaping reasoning. The implicit readiness to aggress is therefore likely to be only modest or indeterminate.

Verbal/Visual Conditional Reasoning Test (VCRT)

For less adept readers, a test based on a "verbal-visual" version of a subset of the CR problems was designed to have a threshold reading level of approximately the fifth to sixth grade (Green & James, 1999). Referred to as the VCRT, this test consists of bare-bones versions of CR problems. The problems are presented both verbally and in written form using a videocassette player and television. The written component consists of simplified prose, which is overlaid on a photograph consistent with the basic theme of the CR problem. The current VCRT contains 14 CR problems, 12 of which are shared with the CRT–A. Work continues on converting CRT–A problems to the VCRT format. Scoring and interpretation of scores on the VCRT are analogous to procedures employed on the CRT–A.

In sum, scores on linear composites of CR problems from either the CRT–A or the VCRT are interpreted in terms of individual differences on the psychological scale labeled CR–A. Individuals with high scores on the CR–A scale are prepared to rationalize aggression and thus are expected to have a significantly greater probability of engaging in aggressive acts than individuals with low or moderate scores on the CR–A scale. The degrees to which scores from the CR–A scale correlate significantly with indicators of aggressive behavior thus become key tests of the scale's empirical and construct validity. Validity coefficients and other relevant evidence for the CR–A scale are summarized later. More complete treatments of psychometric results (e.g., distributions, factor analyses) can be found in the test manual for the CRT–A (James & McIntyre, 2000).

Psychometric Evaluation of CR–A Scale

The following information is presented next:

- Estimates of reliability for scores on the CR–A scale.
- Validities furnished by scores on the CR–A scale.
- Correlations between scores on the CR–A scale and intelligence, gender, and race.
- Correlations between scores on the CR–A scale and self-report measures of aggression.
- Comparative validities for scores from the CR–A scale and self-report measures of aggression.

Much of this information was obtained from the test manual for the CRT–A, although results of recent studies have been added here.

Estimates of Reliability

Three types of reliability were estimated. The set of estimates involved internal consistency estimates (Alpha coefficients) for five factors identified in a factor analysis of the 22 CR problems in the CRT–A. The items factored by JM (i.e., each factor represented one of the JMs in Table 1, with the exception of the Derogation of Target Bias). This factor analysis was conducted on a sample of 1,603 individuals, approximately 50% of whom were college students. The remainder were nonacademic employees. Beginning with Factor 1, the alphas were .87, .82, .81, .76, and .74, respectively. These results suggested that the CR problems associated with each factor provided a reliable estimate of the true score on the JM represented by the factor.

The second type of reliability involved internal consistency estimates for the CR–A scores on the CRT–A and the VCRT. The estimate of reliability for the 22-problem CRT–A was based on the same sample as used in the factor analysis (n = 1,603). A Kuder–Richardson (Formula 20) coefficient (cf. Gulliksen, 1950, Ch. 16, 21) was .76. This value indicates that the total score on the 22-problem CRT–A is a reliable estimate of the true score that would be obtained if all possible CR problems from a heterogeneous domain of CR problems for aggression were answered.

The second internal consistency estimate was obtained for the 14-problem VCRT administered to the 225 college students. The Kuder–Richardson estimate was .78.

The third and final type of reliability was based on a hybrid alternative forms analysis. Undergraduates in one of the first development samples ($n = 276$) were given an early version of a 25-problem CRT for aggression during the first week of a semester. Two months later they were given a VCRT, which at that time had 12 of the 25 CRT problems translated into the VCRT format. Percentage agreement was computed for each of the 12 problems. The values of percentage agreement ranged from 64.9% to 94.6%, with a mean of 81.4%. The estimated correlation between the total score on the 12-problem VCRT and a composite score based on the 12 CRT problems used to construct the VCRT was .82. This correlation, in concert with the estimates of agreement, indicated a reasonable degree of stability in responses to CR problems as well as a reasonable degree of comparability in the scores produced by a CRT format and a VCRT format.

In sum, initial indications are that the scores furnished by CR instruments for aggression are reliable. The estimates of internal consistency cited earlier are comparable to the estimates obtained for a CRT developed to measure achievement motivation (James, 1998).

We now turn to the important issue of validity coefficients. Before we present the results of the validation analyses, however, it is necessary to address the criteria for aggression that were used to validate the CR–A scale. It is incumbent on us to demonstrate that the behavioral criteria we used in empirical validation studies—absences, early and often disruptive departure from a job (Iverson & Deery, 2001), theft, misrepresentation of effort (lying), low job performance, unreliability, and (student) conduct violations—are manifestations of aggression.

Behavioral Manifestations of Aggression in the Workplace

Workplace aggression is defined as "any form of behavior by individuals that is intended to harm current or previous coworkers or their organization" (Folger & Baron, 1996, p. 52). The most dramatic manifestations of aggression are violent acts meant to be highly injurious to a target. However, acts such as physical assault and homicide have low base rates and constitute only a fraction of the behaviors that are meant to harm others (cf. Baron & Richardson, 1994; Borum, 1996; Neuman & Baron, 1998). In this regard, Folger and Baron (1996) indicated "some workplace aggression research concentrates on physical forms of assault of an active and direct nature. ... Such assaults have the flavor of high drama, but they *do not adequately represent the full gamut of workplace aggression*. Clearly, additional research should address other forms of aggression, such as the passive and indirect variety" (p. 70, italics added).

Folger and Baron (1996) suggested that one of the reasons that research has failed to devote attention to the passive and indirect forms of aggression is that investigators have "failed to view these behaviors as aggressive" (p. 70). Of particular concern here is that hostile intentions are easily concealed and thus what is truly an aggressive behavior (e.g., theft, not showing up for work) is attributed to nonhostile motives, such as personal gain or laziness. However, the behavior may in fact be intended to harm (e.g., to exact retaliation or revenge for a perceived injustice by impeding productivity or undermining authority; cf. Skarlicki & Folger, 1997) and thus may well be acts of aggression. Neuman and Baron (1998) make this point rather forcefully with respect to a manifestation of aggression they refer to as "obstructionism."

> With respect to obstructionism, people do fail to return phone calls, show up late for meetings, absent themselves from work, and delay action on important matters for reasons totally unrelated to aggression. However, when these acts are motivated by malicious intent (*as may often be the case*), their effects can be quite damaging to individuals and organizations. (p. 399, italics added)

In addition to obstructionism (e.g., unresponsiveness, habitual absenteeism, habitual tardiness, and procrastination), easily concealed, nondramatic forms of passive and/or indirect aggression include early and disruptive attrition, theft, lying, low job performance, unreliability, asocial conduct, subtle sabotage of projects or machinery, vandalism, spreading rumors, and failure to issue timely warnings of impending physical or financial danger (Baron & Richardson, 1994; Buss, 1961; Neuman & Baron, 1998; O'Leary-Kelly, Griffin, & Glew, 1996). Skarlicki and Folger (1997, p. 435) included many of these behaviors in what they designated organizational retaliatory behaviors, (ORBs, which are negative workplace behaviors "used to punish the organization and its representatives in response to perceived unfairness" (see also Greenberg, 1990, 2002). Not only are aggressive individuals more likely to perceive unfairness (Douglas & Martinko, 2001), perhaps because their perceptions are implicitly shaped by JMs such as the Victimization by Powerful Others Bias (James & Mazerolle, 2002), but also they are more likely to experience the emotions of anger, outrage, and resentment that engender the desires to punish; that is, to impose "harmful consequences" or to "respond destructively" toward, which sustain the indirect and covert seeking of retribution (Skarlicki & Folger, 1997).

Most of our criteria (see Table 2) are included in the subset of nondramatic, indirect/passive aggressive behaviors discussed by investigators of workplace aggression. To further support our position that aggression is one of the explanatory constructs underlying our criteria, we turn to recent research on harmful behaviors in the workplace. Of initial concern is research on "deviant workplace behavior," which Bennett and Robinson (2000, p. 349) defined as "voluntary behavior that violates significant organizational norms and, in so doing, *threatens the well-being* of the organization or its members, or both" (italics added to indicate an aggressive component to deviant behavior).

TABLE 2
Uncorrected Validities for Conditional Reasoning–Aggression Scale

Sample No. and Criterion	n	Sample	Instrument	Experimental Design	Uncorrected Validity[a]
1. Supervisory rating—Overall performance	140	Patrol officers	CRT	Concurrent	.49
2. Absences—Lack of class attendance	188	Undergraduates	CRT	Predictive	.37
3. Lack of truthfulness about extra credit	60	Undergraduates	VCRT	Experiment	.49
4. Absences — Lack of work attendance	97	Nuclear facility operators	CRT	Postdictive	.42
5. Student conduct violations	225	Undergraduates	VCRT	Postdictive	.55
6. Attrition	135	Restaurant employees	CRT	Predictive	.32
7. Absences—Lack of work attendance	105	Package handlers	CRT–A	Predictive	.34
8. Work unreliability	111	Temporary employees	CRT–A	Predictive	.43
9. Theft	95	Undergraduates	CRT–A	Experiment	.64
10. Hard fouls and fights in intramural basketball	191	Undergraduates	CRT–A	Predictive	.38

Note. Uncorrected = not corrected for either range restriction or attenuation due to unreliability in either the predictor or the criterion; CRT = Conditional Reasoning Test; concurrent = data were collected at approximately the same time; predictive = data were collected before criterion data; VCRT = Verbal/Visual Conditional Reasoning Test; postdictive = use of archival criterion data to validate a contemporaneous predictor; CRT–A = Conditional Reasoning Test–Aggression.

[a]All correlations are statistically significant, $p < .05$.

Bennett and Robinson (2000) developed two behavioral scales for workplace deviance (organizational deviance and interpersonal deviance). Included among the measures used to construct these scales were criteria that we employed, namely theft, absences, falsification of receipts (lying), and low and unreliable job performance. Lee and Allen (2002, p. 133) indicated that workplace deviance behaviors "are very close to the types of 'aggression' proposed by Buss (1961)." Indeed, Lee and Allen often used deviance and aggression interchangeably.

Hogan and Hogan (1989, p. 273) suggested that a first step in understanding workplace deviance is to identify the construct that is common to "counterproductive acts such as theft, drug and alcohol abuse, lying, insubordination, vandalism, sabotage, absenteeism, and assaultive actions" (p. 273). The common construct proposed by Hogan and Hogan was *organizational delinquency,* which they defined as "antisocial behavior—whose components include *hostility toward authority,* impulsiveness, social insensitivity, and feelings of alienation" (Hogan & Hogan, 1989, p. 277; italics added to indicate presence of aggression). Hogan and Hogan noted further that people who are "unusually *hostile,* insensitive, and alienated quickly (and usually permanently) run afoul of public authority" whereas people who are "only moderately *hostile,* impulsive, insensitive, and alienated" (p. 277; italics added), the more typical case for organizational delinquents, tend to have fewer legal problems but change jobs frequently, do not achieve significantly, engage in theft (but are seldom caught), have excessive absences and tardiness, malinger, cause damage to equipment (by sabotage [indirect aggression] or by lack of maintenance [passive aggression]), file an inordinate amount of grievances, are insubordinate, and break rules. In sum, aggression is a cause of organizational delinquency and indicators of organizational delinquency include many of the behaviors that we used as criteria (e.g., absences, theft, lying, conduct violations).

Finally, our criteria can be linked to aggression via studies of (a) *counterproductive performance,* which is defined as "voluntary behavior that *harms the well-being* of the organization" and includes behaviors such as absences, theft, and low productivity (Rotundo & Sackett, 2002, p. 69; italics added); and (b) *dysfunctional resistance tactics,* which consist of *passive-aggressive behaviors* such as acting like one did not hear a request (Tepper, Duffy, & Shaw, 2001, p. 975). Of additional relevance is a study by Pearson (1998) that suggested fear of punishment may inhibit direct aggressive actions. Perceived injustice and anger, however, engender retaliation in terms of what Pearson (1998, p. 204) referred to as "displaced aggression." The idea of displacement is to transfer the taking of retribution to a less powerful target, which in this case manifests as attempting to harm the organization (e.g., disrupting organized and planned activities, impeding productivity,) by engaging in passive-aggressive behaviors such as absenteeism, tardiness, and turnover (especially early withdrawal).

In sum, aggression is an intrinsic component of workplace deviance, organizational delinquency, organizational retribution, counterproductive performance, dysfunctional resistance tactics, obstructive behaviors, and displaced aggression.

This is because many if not most deviant, delinquent, retaliatory, counterproductive, dysfunctionally resistant, obstructive, and displaced behaviors involve intentionally hostile attempts to harm an organization or its constituents by exacting retribution, revenge, and retaliation in ways that disrupt work schedules, impede productivity, weaken morale, undermine authority, encourage rebelliousness, and "get even" with a boss or coworkers (James, 1998). To avoid punishment, these processes seldom involve outright violence or acts that are easily detectable as aggression. Rather, they focus on indirect, passive-aggressive behaviors such as failing to come to work or coming to work late; stealing from those they see as guilty of injustices (to exact restitution); lying to authority figures (to regain face and obtain retribution for being disrespected); and performing in poor, unreliable, or improper manners.

The preceding discussion indicates that it is reasonable to regard habitual absences, low performance, theft, early and disruptive attrition, lying, unreliability, and poor conduct as behavioral indicators of aggression. There is no claim that aggression is the only latent construct underlying these behaviors or that these behaviors exhaust the domain of aggression. Nonetheless, these behaviors have often been used as indicators of workplace aggression, and should suffice as "important external variables" (Ozer, 1999) on which to conduct the initial validation studies for the CR measure of aggression.

Results of 10 Empirical Validation Studies

Results of empirical validation studies conducted on 10 separate samples are presented in Table 2. These results indicated that the higher the score on the CR–A scale, the greater the likelihood of engaging in a behavioral manifestation of aggression. Specifically, individuals whose scores indicated that JMs for aggression were instrumental in shaping reasoning had significantly greater probabilities of engaging in aggressive acts than individuals whose scores indicated that JMs were not instrumental in reasoning. For example, college undergraduates with comparatively higher scores on the CR–A scale were more likely than students with lower scores to have committed a student conduct violation ($r = .55$), to have misrepresented (i.e., been untruthful about) the extra-credit points they deserved for participating in an experiment ($r = .49$), to have been absent from class ($r = .37$), to steal when frustrated ($r = .64$), and to have committed acts of physical violence in intramural basketball games ($r = .38$).

Patrol officers with higher CR–A scores were more likely than patrol officers with lower scores to have poor performance ratings ($r = -.49$). Temporary workers with the higher scores were more likely to be unreliable ($r = .43$), whereas nuclear facility operators and package handlers with the higher scores were more likely to be absent from work ($rs = .42$ and $.34$, respectively). Finally, new restaurant employees with the higher CR–A scores were more likely to quit within 30 days of being hired ($r = .32$).

The average validity of the 10 studies in Table 2 is .44. If we were to follow current convention and correct .44 for such things as unreliability in the criterion and range restriction in the predictor (cf. Schmidt & Hunter, 1998), then the .44 could surpass .60, depending on the assumptions used for corrections. However, the observed values in Table 2 reflect what can be expected practically in regard to the use of the CR–A scale in applications such as selection and placement.

The magnitudes of the empirical validities, which were all based on a priori scoring or cross-validation, also deserve brief mention. To put a mean validity of .44 in perspective, consider that uncorrected empirical validities for single predictors against behavioral criteria rarely exceed .40 for aptitude measures and .30 for (primarily self-report) personality measures (cf. Barrick & Mount, 1991, 1993; Ghiselli, 1966; Hough, 1992; Hough, Eaton, Dunnette, Kamp, & McCloy, 1990; Hurtz & Donovan, 2000; Mischel, 1968; Salgado, 1997; Schmitt, Gooding, Noe, & Kirsch, 1984; Tett, Jackson, & Rothstein, 1991). The mean of .44 indicates that the CR–A scale is capable of generating validities of comparatively substantial magnitudes for single, psychological predictors.

Correlations Between Scores on the CR–A Scale and Critical Intellectual Skills

Correlations between scores on the CR–A scale and critical intellectual skills are presented in Table 3. These statistics are reported for three samples of undergraduates. Measurement of critical intellectual skills was based on scores from tests developed by American College Testing (ACT scores). Scores were obtained from student records after obtaining informed consent from the students.

Of initial note is that there is no theoretical reason to expect a correlation between CR for aggression and intelligence. If a correlation were observed, then critical intellectual skills might in some way be confounded with responses to the CR problems. For example, NA alternatives might in some rational way, perceptible by intelligent respondents, be "more logical" than the AG alternatives. However, the correlations in Table 3 indicated that no such confounding took place. Critical intellectual skills were not significantly correlated with the scores on the CR–A scale.

TABLE 3
Correlations Between Scores on Conditional Reasoning–Reasoning Scale
and Critical Intellectual Skills

Study	Intelligence Scale	n	Sample	Correlation
2	ACT	188	Undergraduates	−.06
3	ACT	60	Undergraduates	−.05
5	ACT	225	Undergraduates	−.08

Note.   ACT = American College Testing.

Correlations Between Scores on the CR–A Scale and Gender and Race

Correlations between scores on the CR–A scale and gender are presented in Section A of Table 4. Relations with race are presented in Section B of the same table. Statistics involving gender are presented for the seven samples from the 10 empirical validity studies that included a reasonably large proportion of women (.25 or greater). Statistics for race are presented for the four samples from this set for which race data were available and the proportion of respondents in the largest minority group was .04 of the total sample or greater.

Scores on the CR–A scale did not correlate significantly with gender in five of the seven samples, which included both academic and working groups. Small but significant correlations were obtained in two academic samples. These are

TABLE 4
Relations Between Scores on Conditional Reasoning–Aggression
Scale and Gender and Race

A. Correlations With Gender (Men = 0, Women = 1)				
Sample	Composition	Proportion Women	Point Biserial Correlation	Biserial Correlation
2	188 undergraduates	.34	−.08	−.10
3	60 undergraduates	.60	−.22*	−.29*
5	225 undergraduates	.49	−.20*	−.25*
6	120 restaurant employees	.66	−.06	−.08
7	105 package handlers	.26	.04	.05
8	111 temporary employees	.36	.07	.09
9	95 undergraduates	.55	.00	.00

B. Relations With Race				
Sample	Composition	Proportion	Race	Relationship
2	188 undergraduates	.90	White (0)	$r = .06$[a]
		.10	African American (1)	$(r = .10)$[b]
7	105 package handlers	.23	White	$F = 1.43$
		.52	African American	
		.24	Hispanic	
		.01	Asian	
8	111 temporary employees	.82	White (0)	$r = .07$
		.18	African American (1)	$(r = .10)$
9	95 undergraduates	.57	White	$F = .16$
		.38	Asian	
		.04	Hispanic	
		.01	African American	

[a]Point biserial correlation. [b]Biserial correlation.
*$p < .05$.

point-biserial correlations. This estimator was used because gender is a true dichotomy. On the other hand, the biserial correlation is the more accurate estimator when p values depart from .50 (Lord & Novick, 1968). Thus, biserial correlations are also reported in Table 4. There were no inconsistencies in the statistical inferences based on the two estimators. Both sets of correlations indicated a tendency for young, adult, educationally motivated men to have slightly higher scores than young, adult, educationally motivated women. This tendency was not consistent across all undergraduate samples and did not extend to more intellectually heterogeneous samples. In all, a generally low and nonsignificant correlation between gender and the CR–A scale is indicated.

Race was unrelated to the scores on the CR–A scale. The nonsignificant biserial/point-biserial correlations in Samples 2 and 8 indicated that mean scores on the CR–A scale did not differ significantly between African Americans and Whites. The nonsignificant F tests in Samples 7 and 9 had similar implications (a t test between Whites and African Americans in Sample 7 was also nonsignificant). There was thus no indication that members of different races were more or less implicitly prepared to aggress.

Relations Between Scores on the CR–A Scale and Self-Report Measures of Aggression

Self-report measures of conscious (explicit) cognitions have a history of low and often nonsignificant correlations with various measures, typically projective, of implicit cognitions (Greenwald & Banaji, 1995; McClelland, Koestner, & Weinberger, 1989). Bornstein (2002) recently reviewed this literature and concluded that:

> A paradox has emerged in contemporary personality research. This paradox—which might usefully be termed the *heteromethod convergence problem*—is as follows: Even when self-report and projective measures of a given trait, motive, or need state both predict theoretically related features of behavior, scores on the two tests correlate modestly with each other. (p. 47)

This pattern of modest relations between explicit and implicit measures extended to scores on the CR–A scale (see Table 5). (CR is considered projective in the sense that JMs are implicitly mapped or "projected" into reasoning; James, 1998.) Scores on the CR–A scale shared no more, and typically less than, 7% of their variance with self-ascriptions of aggression from recognized self-report personality inventories (dutifulness in Sample 5 was expected to be an indicator of low aggressiveness). Based on Bornstein's (2002) review, the likely reason for these modest relations is not, as psychometricians have mistakenly thought over the years, lack of convergent validity. Rather, self-reports and projective techniques measure complementary (i.e., explicit and implicit) aspects of traits, motives, biases, and

TABLE 5
Correlations Between Scores on Conditional Reasoning–Aggression
Scale and Self-Report Measures of Aggression

Sample	Composition	Alternative Measure	Correlation
3	60 undergraduates	PRF Aggression	.14
		PRF Dominance	.05
		PRF Impulsivity	.11
5	225 undergraduates	NEO–PI–R Angry Hostility	.26*
		NEO–PI–R Dutifulness	–.18*
9	95 undergraduates	Aggression Questionnaire	.24*
10	191 undergraduates	NEO–PI–R Angry Hostility	.002

Note. PRF = Personality Research Form (Jackson, 1967); NEO–PI–R = Revised NEO Personality Inventory (Costa & McCrae, 1992); Aggression Questionnaire (Buss & Perry, 1992).
  *$p < .05$.

need states. There is no simple pattern to how these explicit and implicit components relate. Indeed, the explicit and implicit facets may conflict, one may compensate for the other, they may work in harmony, or they may work independently—it depends on the constructs and the people.

This is clearly an issue for future research. Readers are referred to excellent new theories regarding interfaces between explicit and implicit measurements in Bornstein (2002; process dissociation models) and Winter et al. (1998; channeling models).

A related issue raised by several reviewers is: What would be the relation between scores on the CR–A scale and scores obtained by simply asking respondents to describe their use of JMs on self-report items? To answer this question, we recently designed a 21-problem self-report instrument on which respondents described the degree to which assumptions or conclusions engendered by the JMs in Table 1 applied to them. An illustrative item for the Victimization by Powerful Others Bias is "I feel that I often get taken advantage of in life" on a scale ranging from 1 (*strongly disagree*) to 5 (*strongly agree*). Based on a sample of 337 undergraduates, the correlation between scores on the CR–A scale and a composite score based on the 21 self-report items was .17 ($p < .01$). Although significant, this correlation indicates that explicit attempts to measure implicit biases accounts for less than 3% of the variance in the implicit measures. Basically, these results support the theory underlying the development of the CRT–A, which is that people cannot introspect and accurately describe their implicit biases.

Multiple Regression and Dominance Analyses

Table 6 reports results of multiple regression analyses (Multiple R, Zero-Order Correlations, and Beta Weights), which regressed behavioral criteria on the CR–A scale and the self-report measures (and ACT scores in Study 3) and dominance

TABLE 6
Multiple Regression-Dominance Analyses

Sample	Criterion	Multiple R	Variable	Zero-Order r	Beta Weight	Relative Importance
3	Lack of truthfulness about extra credit	.55*	CR–A	.49*	.51*	82.83%
			ACT	−.07	−.12	2.89%
			PRF Aggression	.16	.17	8.11%
			PRF Impulsiveness	.14	.14	6.05%
			PRF Dominance	.05	.04	.72%
5	Student conduct violations	.61*	CR–A	.55*	.53*	77.60%
			NEO Angry Hostility	.26*	.21*	16.00%
			NEO Dutifulness	−.18*	−.13*	6.43%
9	Theft	.70*	CR–A	.64*	.57*	71.7%
			Aggression Questionnaire	.44*	.30*	28.3%
10	Hard fouls and fights	.45*	CR–A	.38*	.38*	74%
			NEO Angry Hostility	.22*	.22*	26%

Note. CR–A = Conditional Reasoning–Aggression Scale; ACT = American College Testing; PRF = Personality Research Form; NEO = Personality Inventory (Revised).
*$p < .05$.

analyses (Relative Importance) for the four samples from Table 5. By way of brief explanation, dominance analysis estimates the "relative importance of the p predictors in a specific model" (Budescu, 1993, p. 549). These relative importance values can be interpreted as the proportion or percentage that a particular variable contributes to the R^2. For example, in Study 3, the proportional contribution of the CR–A scale to prediction (i.e., to R^2) was approximately 83%. The Personality Research Form-based self-report of aggression had approximately an 8% proportional contribution to prediction. Thus, of these two predictors, the CR–A scale was the more important.

The findings of the dominance analyses denote that the CR–A scale was relatively more important (i.e., contributed a greater percentage to the R^2) than the self-report measures in predicting lack of truthfulness about extra credit in Sample 3, student conduct violations in Sample 5, theft in Sample 9, and physical violence in basketball in Sample 10. The CR–A scale was also relatively more important than critical intellectual skills (ACT scores) in predicting the truthfulness criterion. The self-report measures split over samples in regard to whether they had significant validities against the criteria. In every case, however, the proportional contribution made by the CR–A scale to the R^2 was greater, typically substantially so, than the self-report measures.

Conclusions and Comments Regarding Psychometric Results

A fair conclusion would seem to be that the CR–A scale offers a valid, efficient, and indirect system for measuring whether JMs are instrumental in shaping reasoning. The presence of JMs in the implicit cognitive system indicates a propensity to engage in aggression in the future. This suggests that evaluators may wish to consider supplementing the traditional self-report items for aggression with CR problems. Results of the multiple regression and dominance analyses indicate that the addition of CR problems will significantly if not substantially increase the capacity to predict whether respondents will behave aggressively in the future.

Questions have arisen regarding what respondents think of the CR problems. An analysis of the verbal protocols of subjects completing CR problems indicated that interviewees believed they were completing reasoning problems. Experience with thousands of administrations of (V)CRTs (which includes CRTs for achievement motivation) also suggests that respondents generally believe that they have completed a test of reasoning skills. Interestingly, a number of respondents have inquired about their scores and several instances of cheating have occurred in which a respondent copied the answer sheet of another respondent.

CONCLUDING COMMENTS

Guion and Gottier (1965) and Guion (1965) engendered considerable consternation about personality testing in organizations with their conclusion that there was little predictive validity in personality test scores. A well-thought-of text in psychometrics proclaimed that the major source of variance in self-report measurements of personality is social desirability (Nunnally, 1967). The ensuing period of 20 or so years is aptly captured by Goldberg's (1993, p. 1) statement: "Once upon a time, we had no personalities." Goldberg went on to say that "Fortunately, times change..." The resurgence of interest in personality in organizational research is documented by many recent contributions, including an article entitled "Rumors of the Death of Dispositional Research are Vastly Exaggerated" by House, Shane, and Herold (1996).

Yet, it is also true that recent meta-analyses have reported that the average, uncorrected validity between self-descriptions of personality and salient, naturally occurring behavioral (performance) criteria is approximately .12, with a maximum rarely exceeding .30 (cf., Barrick & Mount, 1991; Schmitt, Gooding, et al., 1984; Tett, Jackson, & Rothstein, 1991). (A recent review by Schmidt and Hunter, 1998, declined to report uncorrected coefficients.) This same conclusion was reached by Mischel (1968) based on a review of general personality at that time. What has happened in the intervening 30 years to enhance the validity of personality measures? The answer with respect to self-report measures is that instruments such as the revised California Personality Inventory, the Hogan Personality Inventory, and the NEO Personality Inventory (Revised) are improved self-report measures. However, they are still self-report measures, and the ceiling on validity has changed little.

Thus, in the context of self-reports we believe that it is fair to ask: Are the factors that got personality in trouble in the 1960s still in place now? We submit that the answer would be "yes" if new research had not shown a way to involve self-reports in a more useful and valid measurement paradigm. This system involves new measurement procedures such as that offered by CR. Note that we are not recommending that a moratorium be called on self-report measures. Rather, we are recommending that the scope of personality assessment be broadened to include appraisals of implicit cognitions such as the JMs for aggression measured by CR.

Finally, it is possible to think of how the CR approach might be extended beyond aggression and achievement motivation. This system is theoretically generalizable to any behavior that is subject to justification (rationalization) by at least some individuals. Negative traits such as racism, antisocial actions, dishonesty, exploitation, narcissism, and rigidity are obvious candidates. However, it is also possible to engage in justifications for "positive" behaviors, such as when a search for excellence masks an obsessive quest for perfection, or when social conformity is used to mask submissiveness. Thus, the approach has many potential applications.

REFERENCES

Anderson, E. (1994, May). The code of the streets. *The Atlantic Monthly, 5,* 81–94.

Baron, R. A., & Richardson, D. R. (1994). *Human aggression* (2nd ed.). New York: Plenum.

Barrick, M. R., & Mount, M. K. (1991). The Big Five personality dimensions and job performance: A meta-analysis. *Personnel Psychology, 44,* 1–26.

Barrick, M. R., & Mount, M. K. (1993). Autonomy as a moderator of the relationship between the Big Five personality dimensions and job performance. *Journal of Applied Psychology, 78,* 111–118.

Baumeister, R. F., Smart, L., & Boden, J. M. (1996). Relation of threatened egotism to violence and aggression: The dark side of high self-esteem. *Psychological Review, 103,* 5–33.

Bennett, R. J., & Robinson, S. L. (2000). Development of a measure of workplace deviance. *Journal of Applied Psychology, 85,* 349–360.

Bornstein, R. F. (2002). A process dissociation approach to objective-projective test score interrelationships. *Journal of Personality Assessment, 78,* 47–68.

Borum, R. (1996). Improving the clinical practice of violence risk assessment: Technology, guidelines, and training. *American Psychologist, 51,* 945–956.

Bradbury, T. N., & Fincham, F. D. (1990). Attributions in marriage: Review and critique. *Psychological Bulletin, 107,* 3–33.

Budescu, D. V. (1993). Dominance analysis: A new approach to the problem of relative importance of predictors in multiple regression. *Psychological Bulletin, 114,* 542–551.

Buss, A. H. (1961). *The psychology of aggression.* New York: Wiley.

Buss, A. H., & Perry, M. (1992). The aggression questionnaire. *Journal of Personality and Social Psychology, 63*, 452–459.

Crick, N. R., & Dodge, K. A. (1994). A review and reformulation of social information-processing mechanisms in children's social adjustment. *Psychological Bulletin, 115*, 74–101.

Dodge, K. A. (1986). A social information processing model of social competence in children. In M. Perlmutter (Ed.), *The Minnesota symposium on child psychology* (Vol. 18, pp. 77–125). Hillsdale, NJ: Lawrence Erlbaum Associates, Inc.

Douglas, S. C., & Martinko, M. J., (2001). Exploring the role of individual differences in the prediction of workplace aggression. *Journal of Applied Psychology, 86*, 547–559.

Felson, R. B., & Tedeschi, J. T. (Eds.). (1993). *Aggression and violence: Social interactionist perspectives.* Washington, DC: American Psychological Association.

Folger, R., & Baron, R. A. (1996). Violence and hostility at work: A model of reactions to perceived injustice. In G. R. VandenBos & E. Q. Bulatao (Eds.), *Violence on the job: Identifying risks and developing solutions* (Vol. 2, pp. 51–85). Washington, DC: American Psychological Association.

Galotti, K. M. (1989). Approaches to studying formal and everyday reasoning. *Psychological Bulletin, 105*, 331–351.

Gay, P. (1993). *The cultivation of hatred.* New York: Norton.

Ghiselli, E. E. (1966). *The validity of occupational aptitude tests.* New York: Wiley.

Goldberg, L. R. (1993). The structure of phenotypic personality traits. *American Psychologist, 48*, 26–34.

Green, P. D., & James, L. R. (1999, May). The use of conditional reasoning to predict deceptive behavior. In L. J. Williams & S. M. Burroughs (Chairs), *New developments using conditional reasoning to measure employee reliability.* Symposium presented at the meeting of the Society for Industrial and Organizational Psychology, Atlanta.

Greenberg, J. (1990). Employee theft as a reaction to underpayment inequity: The hidden cost of pay cuts. *Journal of Applied Psychology, 75*, 561–568.

Greenberg, J. (2002). Who stole the money, and when? Individual and situational determinants of employee theft. *Organizational Behavior and Human Decision Processes, 89*, 985–1003.

Greenwald, A. G., & Banaji, M. R. (1995). Implicit social cognition: Attitudes, self-esteem, and stereotypes. *Psychological Review, 102*, 4–27.

Guion, R. M. (1965). *Personality testing.* New York: McGraw Hill.

Guion, R. M., & Gottier, R. F. (1965). Validity of personality measures in personnel selection. *Personnel Psychology, 18*, 135–164.

Gulliksen, H. (1950). *Theory of mental tests.* New York: Wiley.

Hogan, J., & Hogan, R. (1989). How to measure employee reliability. *Journal of Applied Psychology, 74*, 273–279.

Hough, L. M. (1992). The "Big Five" personality variables construct confusion: Description versus prediction. *Human Performance, 5*, 139–155.

Hough, L. M., Eaton, N. K., Dunnette, M. D., Kamp. J. D., & McCloy, R. A. (1990). Criterion-related validities of personality constructs and the effect of response distortion on those validities [Monograph]. *Journal of Applied Psychology, 75*, 581–595.

House, R. J., Shane, S. A., & Herold, D. M. (1996). Rumors of the death of dispositional research are vastly exaggerated. *Academy of Management Review, 21*, 203–224.

Huesmann, L. R. (1988). An information processing model for the development of aggression. *Aggressive Behavior, 14*, 13–24.

Hurtz, G. M., & Donovan, J. J. (2000). Personality and job performance: The Big Five revisited. *Journal of Applied Psychology, 85*, 869–879.

Iverson, R. D., & Deery, S. J. (2001). Understanding the "personological" basis of employee withdrawal: The influence of affective disposition on employee tardiness, early departure, and absenteeism. *Journal of Applied Psychology, 86*, 856–866.

James, L. R. (1998). Measurement of personality via conditional reasoning. *Organizational Research Methods, 1*, 131–163.

James, L. R. & McIntyre, M.D. (2000). *Conditional Reasoning Test of Aggression test manual.* San Antonio, TX: Psychological Corporation. (Also available from Knoxville, TN: Innovative Assessment Technology.)

James, L. R., & Mazerolle, M. D. (2002). *Personality at work.* Beverly Hills, CA: Sage.

James, L. R., & Rentsch, J. R. (in press) J_U_S_T_I_F_Y To explain the reasons why: A conditional reasoning approach to understanding motivated behavior. In B. Schneider & B. Smith (Eds.), *Personality and organizations.* Mahwah, NJ: Lawrence Erlbaum Associates, Inc.

Kuhn, D. (1991). *The skills of argument.* New York: Cambridge University Press.

Laursen, B., & Collins W. A. (1994). Interpersonal conflict during adolescence. *Psychological Bulletin, 115,* 197–209.

Lee, K., & Allen, N. J. (2002). Organizational citizenship behavior and workplace deviance: The role of affect and cognitions. *Journal of Applied Psychology, 87,* 131–142.

Lord, F. M., & Novick, M. R. (1968). *Statistical theories of mental tests.* Reading, MA: Addison-Wesley.

McClelland, D. C., Koestner, R., & Weinberger, J. (1989). How do self-attributed and implicit motives differ? *Psychological Review, 96,* 690–702.

Mischel, W. (1968). *Personality and assessment.* New York: Wiley.

Neuman, J. H., & Baron, R. A. (1998). Workplace violence and workplace aggression: Evidence concerning specific forms, potential causes, and preferred targets. *Journal of Management, 24,* 391–419.

Nisbett, R. E. (1993). Violence and U.S. regional culture. *American Psychologist, 48,* 441–449.

Nisbett, R. E., & Wilson, T. D. (1977). Telling more than we can know: Verbal reports on mental processes. *Psychological Review, 84,* 231–259.

Nunnally, J. C. (1967). *Psychometric theory.* New York: McGraw-Hill.

O'Leary-Kelly, A. M., Griffin, R. W., & Glew, D. J. (1996). Organization-motivated aggression: A research framework. *Academy of Management Review, 21,* 225–253.

Ozer, D. J. (1999). Four principles of personality assessment. In L. A. Pervin & O. P. John (Eds.), *Handbook of personality: Theory and research* (2nd ed., pp. 671–688). New York: Guilford.

Pearson, C. M. (1998). Organizations as targets and triggers of aggression and violence: Framing rational explanations for dramatic organizational deviance. *Sociology of Organizations, 15,* 197–223.

Rotundo, M., & Sackett, P. R. (2002). The relative importance of task, citizenship, and counterproductive performance to global ratings of job performance: A policy-capturing approach. *Journal of Applied Psychology, 87,* 66–80.

Salgado, J. G. (1997). The Five Factor Model of personality and job performance in the European community. *Journal of Applied Psychology, 82,* 30–43.

Schmidt, F. L., & Hunter, J. E. (1998). The validity and utility of selection methods in personnel psychology: Practical and theoretical implications of 85 years of research findings. *Psychological Bulletin, 124,* 262–274.

Schmitt, N., Gooding, R. Z., Noe, R. A., & Kirsch, M. (1984). Meta-analyses of validity studies published between 1964 and 1982 and the investigation of study characteristics. *Personnel Psychology, 37,* 407–422.

Schwarz, N. (1999). Self-reports: How the questions shape the answers. *American Psychologist, 54,* 93–105.

Skarlicki, D. P. & Folger, R. (1997). Retaliation in the workplace: The roles of distributive, procedural, and interaction justice. *Journal of Applied Psychology, 82,* 434–443.

Sternberg, R. J. (1984). Reasoning, problem solving, and intelligence (Chapter 5) in R. J. Sternberg (Ed.), *Handbook of human intelligence* (pp. 227–295). Cambridge, England: Cambridge University Press.

Tedeschi, J. T., & Nesler, M. S. (1993). Grievances: Development and reactions. In R. B. Felson & James T. Tedeschi (Eds.), *Aggression and violence: Social interactionist perspectives* (pp. 13–46). Washington, DC: American Psychological Association.

Tepper, B. J., Duffy, M. K., & Shaw, J. D. (2001). Personality moderators of the relationship between abusive supervision and subordinates' resistance. *Journal of Applied Psychology, 86,* 974–983.

Tett, R. P., Jackson, D. N., & Rothstein, M. (1991). Personality measures as predictors of job performance: A meta-analytic review. *Personnel Psychology, 44,* 703–742.

Toch, H. (1993). Good violence and bad violence: Self-presentations of aggressors through accounts and war stories. In R. B. Felson & J. T. Tedeschi (Eds.), *Aggression and violence: Social interactionist perspectives* (pp. 193–206). Washington, DC: American Psychological Association.

Wagner, R. K., & Sternberg, R. J. (1985). Practical intelligence in real-world pursuits: The role of tacit knowledge. *Journal of Personality and Social Psychology, 49,* 436–458.

Wagner, R. K., & Sternberg, R. J. (1986). Tacit knowledge and intelligence in the everyday world. In R. J. Sternberg & R. K. Wagner (Eds.), *Practical intelligence: Nature and origins of competence in the everyday world* (pp. 51–83). New York: Cambridge University Press.

Winter, D. G., John, O. P., Stewart, A. J., Klohnen, E. C., & Duncan, L. E. (1998). Traits and motives: Toward an integration of two traditions in personality research. *Psychological Review, 105,* 230–250.

Wright, J. C., & Mischel, W. (1987). A conditional approach to dispositional constructs: The local predictability of social behavior. *Journal of Personality and Social Psychology, 53,* 1159–1177.

HUMAN PERFORMANCE, *17*(3), 297–324

Individual Differences in Tolerance for Contradiction

David Chan
Department of Social Work and Psychology
National University of Singapore

This article introduces and provides validity evidence for the new individual difference construct of *tolerance for contradiction*, defined as a mode of thinking that accepts and even thrives on apparent bivalent logical contradictions. In Study 1, which used a sample of 198 undergraduates, convergent and discriminant validity evidence for tolerance for contradiction were obtained via associations with a set of established variables. In Study 2, further validity evidence was obtained and the relevance of tolerance for contradiction in the workplace was demonstrated using a sample of 142 prison officers. Tolerance for contradiction was found to interact with situational judgment ability to affect job performance in the manner as hypothesized. The findings on the nature of the interaction supported the argument that tolerance for thinking may be either adaptive or maladaptive. Limitations and implications of the studies as well as future research directions on the construct of tolerance for contradiction were discussed.

When a problem appears to have two equally effective but opposing solutions, how likely would you think that the problem has been poorly defined or poorly represented? If there is a puzzling issue with two opposing but equally possible interpretations, how likely would you proceed to gather information to rule out one of the two interpretations? What do you think of people who maintain that it is possible for two opposing interpretations of the same event to be both true? Responses to these questions are likely to differ across individuals. These differences in responses are important because they affect the way in which the individual views an issue, interprets an event, and approaches or solves a problem. Differences in the way the issue, event, or problem is handled could in turn affect the effectiveness of

---

Requests for reprints should be sent to David Chan, Department of Social Work and Psychology, National University of Singapore, 10 Kent Ridge Crescent, Singapore 119260, Republic of Singapore. E-mail: davidchan@nus.edu.sg

response behavior or problem solving (i.e., performance), although the direction and strength of the effect are likely to depend on the specific problem and context.

The response to questions such as those stated depends on the extent to which the individual tolerates the apparent bivalent logical contradiction alluded to in the questions. The logical contradiction, syntactically expressed in the form of "A & not-A," is contained in the simultaneous endorsement of two opposing solutions to a problem or two opposing interpretations of an issue/event. Are some individuals more tolerant than others of such contradictions? Put in another way, are some individuals more accepting of these contradictions or even thrive on them? This article's premise is that individuals systematically differ in their level of tolerance for contradiction. The purpose of this article is to introduce and validate the construct of *tolerance for contradiction* (TC) as a thinking style individual difference variable, and the validation efforts include demonstrating the construct's relevance in the workplace. Results from two studies provided preliminary validity evidence for this new construct and demonstrated its positive as well as negative effects on job performance.

There exists an extensive literature on individual difference constructs related to thinking style and information processing (for review, see Rayner & Riding, 1997). As explained in Study 1, there are several individual difference constructs that are conceptually similar to tolerance for contradiction (e.g., *Openness to Experience* [OE], *Tolerance of Ambiguity* [TA]). However, these constructs are distinct and they do not capture the essence of tolerance for contradiction.

This article is organized as follows. First, the definition of the TC construct and its conceptual basis are explicated. Study 1, a basic construct validation effort based on an undergraduate sample, is then reported. The study gathered construct validity evidence via nomological validation using a set of established individual difference variables selected in a theory-driven manner. This is followed by Study 2, which involved a sample of prison officers. The study was conducted to demonstrate the relevance of the construct in influencing job-performance either positively or negatively depending on the individual's situational judgment ability. In addition to demonstrating criterion-related validity, Study 2 showed that TC may be either adaptive or maladaptive. This article ends with a discussion on the implications of the two studies and an agenda for future research on the new individual difference construct.

TOLERANCE FOR CONTRADICTION: DEFINITION AND CONCEPTUAL BASIS

The conceptual basis for the TC construct is provided by a juxtaposition of two systems of logic: Aristotle's classical system of bivalent logic consisting of two distinct and mutually exclusive truth values (True or False) versus Zadeh's (1965) system of fuzzy logic, which is a formal theory of sets that calibrates vagueness. A low level of TC is the psychological equivalence of an adherence to Aristotle's bi-valent logic whereas a high level of TC is the psychological equivalence of an adherence to fuzzy logic. The following sections describe the two systems of logic and link them to the thinking style construct of TC.

Bivalent Logic Versus Fuzzy Logic

A conventional approach to thinking is that of dichotomizing the world into dichotomous opposites. Thus, an answer is either right or wrong, a person is either good or evil, and problems are either solved or unsolved. This dichotomous or binary way of thinking does have its advantages. For example, it simplifies complex stimuli into discrete categories that are more manageable and decreases uncertainty (Kosko, 1993). This dichotomous approach to thinking can be traced back to Aristotle. Aristotle's *law of excluded middle* states that it is necessarily true that things are "either A or not-A." In everyday language, the law of excluded middle is often expressed as "P is either A or B," where B is the opposite or negation of A; that is, B is equal to not-A. According to the law of excluded middle, a statement is either true or false. There are only these two truth values (i.e., true or false) and there are no other truth values in between them. In other words, A and not-A are contradictory and complementary so that they are mutually exclusive and jointly exhaustive. A logically equivalent way to express the law of exclude middle is to state that that an assertion (A) and its negation (not-A) cannot occur or be true at the same time. This logical equivalence of Aristotle's law of excluded middle is known as Aristotle's *law of noncontradiction*.[1]

Thus, an act cannot be both right and wrong, a person cannot be both good and evil, and a problem cannot be both solved and unsolved. To assert that "P is A and not-A" is to commit a bivalent logical contradiction. Within the conceptual definition of the TC construct, a low level on the construct would correspond to (i.e., the psychological equivalence of) a thinking style that adheres to Aristotle's system of bivalent logic and one that dismisses as inappropriate, unrealistic, or maladaptive any endorsement of bivalent logical contradictions. Hence, an individual who is low on TC is a bivalent thinker who would, in response to the three questions posed in the beginning of this article, think that the problem has been poorly defined or poorly represented (first question); proceed to gather information to rule out one of the two interpretations (second question); and consider those who maintain that it is possible for two opposing interpretations of the same event to be both true as illogical, unrealistic, and maladaptive individuals (third question).

---

[1] In formal symbolic logic, each of these two laws is a necessary derivation of the other. Because the two laws are logically equivalent, this article, for the purpose of convenience, arbitrarily uses the law of excluded middle to refer to both the law itself and the law of noncontradiction.

The system of fuzzy logic, in contrast, rejects a reductionistic and clear dichotomous either/or, and black/white view of the world. Thus, an answer can be right and wrong at the same time and problems can be both solved and not solved. An individual who is high on TC views the world as inherently ambiguous rather than consisting of precise dichotomous opposites and accepts as reality the paradox of multivalence and apparent binary logical contradictions. This rejection of a black/white view of the world comes from the central idea in fuzzy logic that all things are best characterized in terms of degrees and are not neatly sorted into distinct categories separated by precise and crisp boundaries. Thus, distance, temperature, friendliness, and all other things are never black or white but are in different shades of gray. Bangkok is *very far* from New York. Monday was *quite cold*. John is *fairly friendly*. Thus, the statement "John is a friendly person" is partially true and partially false. Likewise, the statement "John is an unfriendly person" is partially true and partially false. It is this notion of degrees of truth that allows the high TC thinker to embrace the apparently contradictory statement "John is a friendly and unfriendly person." Because all things are on a sliding scale of degrees, it is often impossible to distinguish members of a category from nonmembers. Things have partial memberships in different categories. The notions of degrees of truth and partial memberships together form the essence of fuzzy logic and led the fuzzy logician to reject Aristotle's law of excluded middle (everything is either A or not-A) and law of noncontradiction (nothing can be both A and not-A). Within the conceptual definition of the TC construct, a high level on the construct would correspond to (i.e., the psychological equivalence of) a thinking style that adheres to the system of fuzzy logic and one that dismisses as inappropriate, unrealistic, or maladaptive any endorsement of bivalent assertions in terms of distinct and mutually exclusive truth values. Hence, an individual who is high on TC is a nonbivalent thinker who would not, in response to the three questions posed in the beginning of this article, think that the problem has been poorly defined or poorly represented (first question) or proceed to gather information to rule out one of the two interpretations (second question), and would consider those who maintain that it is possible for two opposing interpretations of the same event to be both true as realistic and adaptive individuals (third question).

Tolerance for Contradiction, Ambiguity, Certainty, and Probability

To better understand fuzziness and hence TC, we need to relate fuzziness to the concepts of ambiguity and certainty. In addition, fuzzy thinking (i.e., TC) should not be confused with probabilistic thinking.

The literature on fuzzy logic makes the important distinction between fuzziness on one hand and ambiguity in the sense of interpretative uncertainty on the other. In our everyday use of the term, ambiguity is said to exist when there are several equally plausible but mutually exclusive interpretations of a word, object, or situation, and there is uncertainty as to which interpretation is true or correct. The ambiguity, however, is not an inherent property and it can be removed with the availability of more information or elaboration of the context. In the statement "John was murdered at the bank," the ambiguity or uncertainty pertaining to the location of the crime is removed if the statement is made in the context of a description of a bank robbery as opposed to a stroll by the river. Ambiguity is therefore the result of a lack of precision or elaboration and it can be removed or at least reduced when more information is available. With sufficient information, ambiguity is removed and certainty or truth in describing reality is achieved. It is in this sense that we ascribe, in our everyday language, a negative connotation when we describe something as ambiguous.

Fuzziness, on the other hand, does not view ambiguity negatively. Fuzzy thinking (i.e., TC) accepts opposing interpretations as both true at the same time and does not view ambiguity as an uncertainty of interpretation waiting to be removed or reduced with additional information. Certainty already exists in the sense that the ambiguity is construed as an inherent property of reality itself, rather than as an obstacle to the true description of reality. The ambiguity in fuzziness is therefore an inherent property and more information would not rule out one interpretation in favor of the other (hence their responses to the three questions posed in the beginning of this article, as noted earlier).

Just as fuzzy logic is conceptually distinct from probability theory, TC is not to be confused with probabilistic thinking. The difference between fuzziness and probability lies in the treatment of uncertainty. In probability, uncertainty is treated as randomness in the context of the likelihood or prediction of the occurrence of an event. Consider the probability that Event A will occur tomorrow. Even today, we are certain that Event A will either occur or not occur tomorrow. After tomorrow, we will know for certain that Event A did or did not occur. That is, in probability theory, uncertainty refers to the likelihood of the occurrence or nonoccurrence of an event. The occurrence or nonoccurrence of the event, however, is certain. The uncertainty comes only from the fact that we cannot observe today the occurrence or nonoccurrence of the event tomorrow. The occurrence and nonoccurrence of the event is binary in nature and mutually exclusive. In other words, in probabilistic thinking, the description of reality remains clearly dichotomous and adheres strictly to Aristotle's law of excluded middle. An individual who has high TC (i.e., a fuzzy thinker), in contrast, is less concerned with the likelihood of the occurrence or nonoccurrence of Event A. Given that an event in fact occurred, individuals high on TC would accept as reality that some elements of Event A are present in the event but other elements of Event A are absent such that it is perfectly consistent to assert that event A both occurred and did not occur. In reality, there can be no absolute certainty in the assertion that Event A occurred (or did not occur). The only certainty is that Event A partially occurred and partially did not occur.[2]

---

[2]Technical and mathematical treatments of the distinction between fuzzy logic and probability theory are available in Cheeseman (1986), McNeill and Freiberger (1993), and Zadeh (1965, 1980).

Fuzzy logic, as a formal theory of sets that calibrates vagueness, has been successfully applied in electronics, engineering, and a host of industrial processes (e.g., Dubios, Nguyen, Prade, & Segeno, 1999; Pal, 1991). Fuzzy systems, which assume that all things are characterized in terms of degrees with continuously graded truth values, are adaptive because they compute with human linguistic variables instead of crisp, dichotomous, and binary truth-values (Rasiowa, 1993). In psychology, there are also parallel attempts to apply the principles of fuzzy logic in reasoning (Reyna & Brainerd, 1992) and perceptions (Massaro & Cohen, 1993). However, there has been no empirical research that directly examines the concept of fuzzy thinking as an individual difference construct (i.e., TC). Study 1 reports empirical research that gathered basic construct validity evidence for the individual difference construct of TC.

STUDY 1

To obtain convergent and discriminant validity evidence for the TC construct, several established individual difference constructs were included in the validation effort. First, to establish convergent validity, individual difference constructs that should have a moderate correlation with TC because of conceptual similarity were included. Next, individual difference constructs that have no conceptual similarity were also selected to establish discriminant validity. That is, these constructs should have zero or trivial correlation with tolerance for contradiction. Table 1 (see column on predicted relations) presents the predicted relations between TC and these established individual difference constructs. The following paragraphs explicate the rationale for the predicted relations.

Predicted Relations in Assessment of Convergent and Discriminant Validity

Need for Precision (NFP) is defined as a preference for using relatively fine-grained information and engaging in thinking involving fine-grained as opposed to coarse-grained distinctions (Viswanathan, 1997). Contrary to a person high in TC, a person high in NFP perceives ambiguous information as a source of threat or discomfort (Viswanathan, 1997). Thus, a moderately negative association is predicted between TC and NFP.

Personal Need for Structure (PNS) is conceptualized as a need to lead a simple, tightly organized life, both cognitively and behaviorally (Neuberg & Newsom, 1993). High PNS individuals are thus motivated to seek out simple and unambiguous ways of dealing with their worlds (Neuberg & Newsom, 1993, p. 113). Contrary to a person high in TC, a person high in PNS should find uncertain and am-

TABLE 1
Convergent and Discriminant Validation of Tolerance for Contradiction:
Predicted Relations and Summary of Results

Individual Difference Variable	Predicted Relations With Tolerance for Contradiction	Correlation	
Convergent validity			
Need for precision	−	−.25*	(−.32)
Personal need for structure	−	−.22*	(−.27)
Tolerance for ambiguity	+	.29*	(.39)
Openness to experience	+	.24*	(.32)
Discriminant validity			
Neuroticism	0	.06	(.07)
Extraversion	0	−.01	(−.01)
Agreeableness	0	.05	(.06)
Conscientiousness	0	−.19*	(−.23)
Proactive personality	0	−.09	(−.11)
Positive affectivity	0	.08	(.10)
Negative affectivity	0	.12	(.14)
Cognitive ability	0	.02	(.02)
Impression management	0	−.02	(−.03)
Gender	0	−.06	(−.07)
Age	0	−.01	(−.01)

Note. $N = 198$. Values in parentheses represent correlations corrected for attenuation due to unreliability of measures. For gender and age, only the reliability of tolerance for contradiction was used for correction. For all other corrections, reliabilities of both measures being correlated were used. For Cognitive Ability, a reliability of .80 was assumed. An en dash (−) = negative relationship; a zero = no relationship; a plus sign (+) = positive relationship.
*$p < .05$.

biguous situations uncomfortable or even stressful. Thus, a moderately negative association is predicted between TC and PNS.

Tolerance for Ambiguity (TA) refers to an individual's willingness to accommodate or adapt to encounters with unfamiliar, ambiguous, complex, or incongruent cues or ideas (Furnham, 1994; Jonassen & Grabowski, 1993). As explained earlier, the literature on fuzzy logic makes the important conceptual distinction between fuzziness and ambiguity (as used in everyday language) in terms of certainty of reality. The construct of TA focuses on ambiguity as an obstacle to achieving certainty or true description of reality. Fuzziness, on the other hand, focuses on ambiguity as an inherent property of the true description of reality. In the construct of TA, ambiguity is uncertainty. At high levels on the construct of TC (which is based on the concept of fuzzy thinking), ambiguity is certainty (as in the literature on fuzzy logic). In short, TA is conceptually similar to TC in that the notion of ambiguity is central in both constructs. However, whereas individuals high in TA tolerate ambiguity, individuals high in TC embrace ambiguity. Hence, a moderately positive association is predicted between TC and TA. As shown later in the items on the measure of TC, the test content of TC and the test content of TA represent distinct constructs.

Openess to Experience (OE) is one dimension of the well-established Big Five personality structure (Digman, 1990). OE is generally defined as a person's inquisitiveness and need to enlarge and examine experience (Mount & Barrick, 1998). It is also associated with creativity and identity flexibility (Mount & Barrick, 1998). Similar to a person high in tolerance for contradiction, a person with high OE is more likely to cope comfortably with uncertain situations and a changing environment. Thus, a moderately positive association is predicted between tolerance for contradiction and OE.

Other than OE, the rest of the Big Five personality traits, namely Neuroticism (N), Extraversion (E), Agreeableness (A), and Conscientiousness (C), do not share any conceptual similarity with tolerance for contradiction and hence are not expected to be associated with the construct. Neuroticism is the tendency to be anxious or worried and is conceptually similar to Negative Affectivity. Extraversion is associated with energy, sociability, excitement, and stimulation (Mount & Barrick, 1998). The major facets of Agreeableness are trust, straightforwardness, and altruism (Costa & McCrae, 1992). Individuals high in Agreeableness are helpful and well-intentioned whereas those low in Agreeableness are skeptical and cynical. Individuals high in Conscientiousness are organized, systematic, and purposeful.

Proactive Personality (PAP; Bateman & Crant, 1993) refers to a stable dispositional construct that identifies differences among individuals in the extent to which they take action to influence their environment. Individuals high on PAP are relatively unconstrained by situational forces and effect environmental change. They are active in scanning the environment for opportunities, showing initiative, taking action, and persevering until they reach closure by bringing about change. Conversely, people who are not proactive are relatively passive—they react to, adapt to, and are shaped by their environment. Not only has Bateman and Crant's (1993) PAP scale been demonstrated to be differentially associated with the widely accepted Big Five personality traits, it has also been able to predict a number of criterion variables over and above the contribution of the Big Five traits and other relevant predictor variables (Crant, 1995; Crant & Bateman, 2000). A number of other studies have consistently demonstrated the validity of the PAP construct (e.g., Crant, 1996; Kirkman & Rosen, 1999; Parker & Sprigg, 1999). Hence, to widen the scope of personality traits included in the validation, the established PAP (Bateman & Crant, 1993) was included in the study to provide discriminant validity. That is, TC is not expected to be associated with PAP.

Positive Affectivity (PA) and *Negative Affectivity* (NA) are two established affectivity individual difference constructs. PA refers to the extent to which a person feels enthusiastic, active, and alert (Watson, Clark, & Tellegen, 1988). High-PA individuals are in a state of high energy and pleasurable engagement, whereas low-PA individuals are characterized by sadness and lethargy. NA, on the other hand, is a general dimension of subjective distress that subsumes a variety of aversive mood states, including anger, contempt, disgust, guilt, fear, and nervousness (Watson et al., 1988). Research has shown that PA and NA are distinct constructs rather than polar ends of a continuum. Given that TC is a preferred mode of thinking, no association is expected between TC and the two affectivity constructs (PA and NA).

Cognitive Ability (CA) is generally regarded as an individual's capacity, accuracy, and speed of processing information. As a thinking style, TC is an individual's preferred mode of processing information. It is well established that cognitive style and CA (level) are conceptually different (Chan, 1996; Sternberg, 1997; Tucker & Warr, 1996). High TC, as explicated earlier, is a thinking style preference that is the psychological equivalence of an adherence to fuzzy logic (i.e., a rejection of bivalent logic). Individuals with high TC are essentially fuzzy thinkers but they are not equal to individuals with low CA who simply fail to understand bivalent logic. Hence, no association is expected between TC and CA. Finding such an association would be inconsistent with the present conceptual basis for the TC construct.

Impression Management (IM) is a social desirability responding that self-report research often has to deal with. It refers to the deliberate effort to create a specific effect desired by a respondent (Paulhus, 1984). Because TC is a preference mode that individuals themselves ascribe to and social desirability is not inherent in the construct, a valid measure of TC should not be associated with IM.

Finally, there are no theoretical reasons to expect TC to be associated with either gender or age.

Method

Participants and procedure.   A total of 198 undergraduates (51% women) at a large university in Singapore voluntarily participated in this study, receiving $15 for their participation. The mean age of participants was 21.51 years (SD = .92). Participants completed all measures in groups of about 15 in classroom settings. They were told that the purpose of this study was to examine problem-solving styles. All participants were debriefed.

Measures.   TC was measured using the Tolerance for Contradiction Scale (TCS) developed by the author. The TCS is a 10-item measure with a Likert-type rating response format. The items on the TCS were developed from selected items on the 20-item pilot version of the biodata-type measure reported in Chan and Sim (2002). In the pilot version of the measure, the items were of a multiple-choice format; for each item, participants were required to answer a question by choosing from two to five options the one that best describes their past experiences and behaviors. Each item was scored dichotomously (0 and 1). A problem with the pilot version of the measure was its relatively low internal consistency estimate of reliability and low variance accounted for by a single factor solution in a principal components analysis, probably due to the dichotomous nature of item scoring. Hence, in developing the TCS, the multiple-choice format items in the pilot version of the measure were adapted to a typical personality inventory-type format where respondents were simply required to rate, using a 5-point Likert-type rating scale ranging from 1(*strongly disagree*) to 5 (*strongly agree*), the extent to which they agree that a given statement is descriptive of the way they typically approach or solve problems. In the initial development, a total of 14 such items that appeared nonredundant were adapted. In adapting the items, item writing was guided by operationalizing TC in terms of the adherence or nonadherence to notions indicative of Aristotle's law of excluded middle.

Two psychology graduate students, who were earlier briefed by the author on the conceptual definition of the TC construct, independently examined each item to assess their content validity and remove redundant items. Both raters were in complete agreement in removing three items due to redundancy and one item due to unclear item content. Hence, the final measure of TC, which was administered in both Study 1 and Study 2, consisted of 10 items. The complete TCS is presented in the Appendix.

NFP was measured using a 13-item scale developed by Viswanathan (1997). It has a documented Cronbach's alpha of .80 and test–retest reliability (over a 1-week period) of .72. An example item is "I enjoy tasks that require me to be exact." Participants rated the degree of their agreement on a 5-point Likert-type scale ranging from 1 (*strongly disagree*) to 5 (*strongly agree*). Psychometric properties of the measure and evidence of their criterion-related and construct validity are available in Viswanathan (1997).

PNS was measured using the 11-item scale developed by Neuberg and Newsom (1993). The scale has a documented median Cronbach's alpha of .77 and test–retest reliability (over a 12-week period) of .76. An example item is "I enjoy having a clear and structured mode of life." Participants rated the degree of their agreement on a 5-point Likert-type scale ranging from 1 (*strongly disagree*) to 5 (*strongly agree*). Psychometric properties of the measure and evidence of their criterion-related and construct validity are available in Neuberg and Newsom (1993).

TA was measured using the 7-item job-related ambiguity scale developed by Norton (1975). It has a documented Cronbach's alpha of .69 and test–retest reliability of .86 (10–12 weeks). An example item is "I don't like to work on a problem unless there is a possibility of coming out with a clear-cut and unambiguous answer." Participants rated the degree of their agreement on a 5-point Likert-type scale ranging from 1 (*strongly disagree*) to 5 (*strongly agree*). Validity evidence for the measure is available in Ashford and Cummings (1985) and Jonassen and Grabowski (1993).

The Big Five personality traits of Neuroticism (N), Extraversion (E), Openness to Experience (OE), Agreeableness (A) and Conscientiousness (C) were measured using the NEO Five-Factor Inventory (NEO–FFI; Costa & McCrae, 1992). Cronbach's alphas of five scales are reported in the NEO–FFI manual (Costa & McCrae, 1992). Participants rated the degree of their agreement on a 5-point Likert-type scale ranging from 1 (*strongly disagree*) to 5 (*strongly agree*). Psychometric properties of the NEO–FFI and evidence of their criterion-related and construct validity are available in Costa and McCrae (1992) and Digman (1990).

PAP was assessed using the shortened version of Bateman and Crant's (1993) Proactive Personality Scale, developed by Seibert, Crant, and Kraimer (1999) with a reported Cronbach's alpha of .86. Example items on the 10-item measure include "If I see something I don't like, I fix it," "I am always looking for better ways to do things," and "If I believe in an idea, no obstacles will prevent me from making it happen." Responses were indicated on a 7-point scale ranging from 1 (*strongly disagree*) to 7 (*strongly agree*). Items were averaged to arrive at a PAP score. Cronbach's alpha in this study was .92.

PA and NA were measured using a 20-item scale developed by Watson et al. (1988). The PA scale consists of 10 adjectives describing positive feelings and emotions (e.g., interested, active) and the NA scale consists of 10 adjectives describing negative feelings and emotions (e.g., distressed, afraid). Documented Cronbach's alphas for PA and NA are .88 and .87, respectively. Test–retest reliabilities are .68 and .71, respectively, for PA and NA. Participants rated the extent to which they experience the feeling *in general* on a 5-point Likert-type scale ranging from 1 (*very slightly*) to 5 (*very much*). Psychometric properties of the measure and evidence of their criterion-related and construct validity are available in Watson et al. (1988).

Participants' Grade Point Average (GPA), obtained from the university administration with their permission, was used as a proxy measure of CA. The theoretical range for GPA in this university is 0 to 5 points.

IM was measured using the 8-item scale that Chan (2001) adapted from the IM scale developed by Paulhus (1988). It has a documented Cronbach's alpha of .87 and test–retest reliability (over a 10-week period) of .84. An example item is "I sometimes try to get even rather than forgive and forget." Participants rated the degree of their agreement on a 5-point Likert-type scale ranging from 1 (*very true*) to 5 (*very untrue*). Items were dichotomously scored and summed to represent the level of IM, with high scores indicating high IM (see Paulhus, 1988). Psychometric properties and validity evidence for the measure are available in Chan (2001) and Paulhus (1988).

Data analyses.   Principal component analyses and confirmatory factor analyses were used to test the hypothesized one-factor structure of the TCS. Correlational analyses, including both observed correlations and correlations corrected for attenuation due to unreliability, were used to assess convergent and discriminant validity (see Table 1).

Results and Discussion

Principal component analysis performed on the 10 items on the TCS clearly indicated a one-factor solution, as indicated by the scree plot. The single factor accounted for 40% of the total variance. The confirmatory factor analysis showed that a single factor model provided a good fit to the data, as indicated by a convergence of good fit from the various established model fit indexes (nonnormed fit index [NNFI] = .92; comparative fit index [CFI] = .94; standardized root mean square residual [SRMR] = .06; root mean square error of approximation [RMSEA] = .09). All standardized factor loadings were significant ($p < .05$) and of substantial magnitude ranging from .51 to .63 with a mean loading of .57. Hence, there was substantial evidence that the TCS was unitary so that it was meaningful to use the means of the 10 items as a composite score to represent TC. Cronbach's alpha of the measure was .83.

The descriptive statistics of all study variables are presented in Table 2. Table 1 presents the correlations (observed and corrected) between TC and individual difference variables examined in the nomological validation process. As shown in Table 1 (see column on correlations), results confirmed the predicted relations as shown in the same table. As predicted, TC was negatively correlated with NFP ($r = -.25$, $p < .05$) and PNS ($r = -.22$, $p < .05$) and positively correlated with TA ($r = .29$, $p < .05$) and OE ($r = .24$, $p < .05$). Although significant, these correlations were modest in magnitude indicating that the four constructs (NFP, PNS, TA, OE) are distinct from TC.

As expected, TC was not significantly associated with the personality traits of Neurotcism ($r = .06$), Extraversion ($r = -.01$), Agreeableness ($r = .05$), PAP ($r = -.09$), affective dispositions (PA, $r = .08$, NA, $r = .12$), or CA ($r = .02$). There was no evidence of social desirability responding on the measure of TC, as suggested by the absence of correlation between the TC and IM scale ($r = -.02$). As expected, there was no sex difference in TC ($r = -.06$, Cohen's $d = .08$) and the construct was not correlated with age ($r = -.01$). Only 1 of the 15 predicted relations presented in Table 1 was not supported. TC has a significant negative correlation with Conscientiousness, although no association was expected ($r = -.19$, $p < .05$). However, the magnitude of the unexpected significant association is relatively small.

As shown in Table 1, the pattern of corrected correlations mirrored the pattern of observed correlations, indicating that the observed pattern of correlations could not be attributed to differential reliabilities across measures. Overall, the correlational results provided adequate convergent and discriminant validity evidence supporting TC as a distinct construct in the nomological network.

TABLE 2
Means, Standard Deviations, Reliabilities, and Correlations of Study 1 Variables

Variable	M	SD	1	2	3	4	5	6	7	8	9	10	11	12	13	14	15	16
1. TC	3.32	.62	(.83)															
2. NFP	3.34	.45	-.25*	(.72)														
3. PNS	3.00	.59	-.22*	.03	(.82)													
4. TA	2.88	.54	.29*	.02	-.53*	(.67)												
5. OE	3.53	.45	.24*	.21*	-.40*	.22*	(.67)											
6. N	2.56	.56	.06	-.27*	.26*	-.27*	-.12*	(.83)										
7. E	3.63	.49	-.01	.22*	-.30*	.21*	.17*	-.48*	(.80)									
8. A	3.64	.43	.05	.10	-.13*	.22*	.08	-.31*	.29*	(.71)								
9. C	3.75	.51	-.19*	.43*	.31*	-.08	-.01	-.40*	.23*	.17*	(.85)							
10. PAP	5.30	.68	-.09	.38*	-.01	.05	.32*	-.26*	.43*	-.01	.46*	(.82)						
11. PA	3.93	.58	.08	.17*	-.09	-.17*	.12*	-.38*	.45*	.16*	.28*	.46*	(.74)					
12. NA	1.98	.63	.12	-.21*	.09	-.13*	-.01	.51*	-.19*	-.23*	-.29*	-.18*	-.14*	(.88)				
13. CA	3.70	.60	.02	-.03	.05	-.07	-.04	.01	-.11*	-.02	.11	.04	-.10	-.05	—			
14. IM	1.61	1.53	-.02	-.12*	-.14*	.06	.13*	.19*	-.04	-.19*	-.21*	-.05	-.05	.28*	.03	(.55)		
15. Sex	.50	.50	-.06	-.05	.13*	.01	-.08	-.02	-.13*	.02	-.04	.02	.01	.04	.21*	.05	—	
16. Age	21.51	.92	-.01	-.08	-.02	-.08	.07	-.02	.01	-.06	-.05	.09	.04	.02	.10	.10	.48*	—

Note. N = 198. Values in parentheses represent reliabilities obtained in this study. TC = Tolerance for Contradiction; NFP = Need for Precision; PNS = Personal Need for Structure; TA = Tolerance for Ambiguity; OE = Openness to Experience; N = Neuroticism; E = Extraversion; A = Agreeableness; C = Conscientiousness; PAP = Proactive Personality; PA = Positive Affectivity; NA = Negative Affectivity; CA = Cognitive Ability; IM = Impression Management.
*p < .05.

309

The results of Study 1, which were based on an undergraduate sample, provided promising preliminary evidence of construct validity for TC. To obtain further validity evidence for the construct, Study 2, which involved a sample of prison officers, was conducted to demonstrate the relevance of the construct in influencing job performance either positively or negatively depending on the individual's situational judgment ability. In addition to demonstrating criterion-related validity, a major purpose of Study 2 was to show that TC may be either adaptive or maladaptive.

STUDY 2

The purpose of Study 2 was twofold. First, this study provided an actual employee sample to replicate the one-factor structure and reliability of the TCS. To provide a more rigorous cross-validation of the measure, an assessment of measurement invariance of TCS responses between the undergraduate sample in Study 1 and the employee sample in this study was also conducted. Second, the study aimed to demonstrate the relevance of the TC construct in the workplace involving actual employees by showing that TC may be either adaptive or maladaptive. This was accomplished by demonstrating an interaction between TC and situational judgment ability (SJA) in affecting job performance. Demonstrating that TC is neither inherently adaptive nor maladaptive but that it may be either adaptive or maladaptive is important. As noted later, it would help clarify the construct and provide a useful point of departure for future research. This study also provided an opportunity to demonstrate that TC is conceptually and empirically distinct from SJA, by assessing the correlation between the two variables and showing the differential relation with job performance. To achieve the second aim of this study, two hypotheses were formulated and tested. The following paragraphs explicate the rationale for the hypotheses.

SJA, sometimes used interchangeably with the concept of practical intelligence or tacit knowledge, refers to an individual's ability to make an accurate judgment about various aspects of the situation and respond effectively to the practical situational demands (Chan & Schmitt, 2002, McDaniel, Morgeson, Finnegan, Campion, & Braverman, 2001; Sternberg, Wagner, & Okagaki, 1993; Wagner & Sternberg, 1985). For accurate judgment and effective responses to be possible, the individual would need to attend to the relevant content features or cues of the situation and disregard irrelevant ones. Situational judgment tests have been consistently shown to predict job performance and there is increasing evidence that they provide significant incremental prediction over traditional measures of CA, personality, technical job knowledge, and work experience (e.g., Chan & Schmitt, 2002; Clevenger, Pereira, Wiechmann, Schmitt, & Harvey, 2001).

Some may argue that the ability to tolerate contradictions is simply a facet of the more global ability to make accurate and effective situational judgments. If this is true, then we would expect TCS scores to be positively and highly correlated with scores on a test of SJA. On the other hand, others may argue that tolerating contradiction is in fact a manifestation of the failure to recognize contradictions, which is simply a reflection of low ability in one facet of situational judgment. If this is true, then we would expect TCS scores to be negatively and highly correlated with SJA test scores. However, SJA is conceptually distinct from the conceptual definition of the TC construct as explicated earlier. Hence, in this study, no correlation was expected between TC and SJA. This lack of an empirical association would provide further evidence of discriminant validity for the TC construct. Unlike the SJA construct, the conceptual definition of the TC construct is not inherently adaptive or maladaptive with respect to job performance. Hence, unlike SJA, we would not expect a correlation between TC and job performance. Obtaining differential relations with job performance would provide further evidence that TC is distinct from and not a facet of SJA. It is predicted that:

H1:   Situational Judgment Ability (SJA) will positively predict job performance but there will be no association between Tolerance for Contradiction (TC) and job performance.

The tendency to tolerate contradictions in a work situation is likely to be adaptive in terms of job performance when the individual is high on SJA. As noted by many researchers, many situations in today's rapidly changing workplace are dynamic, containing problems that are ill-defined and ambiguous, with no clear cut or categorical answers (Chan, 2000; Pulakos, Arad, Donovan, & Plamondon, 2000). Individuals high on SJA are able to recognize the relevant situational features or cues that represent dynamic aspects in a work situation when they do in fact occur and therefore also more likely to recognize the existence of problem interpretations that are opposing but apparently equally plausible as well as proposed solutions that are opposing but appear to be equally effective. These individuals would often find themselves in contradictory situations confronted with opposing interpretations, solutions, and choices. Among these individuals (i.e., individuals high on SJA), they differ in their tolerance of contradiction. Those who are more tolerant of contradictions would approach or solve the problem in a manner that is consistent with the contradictory nature of the problem, accepting or even thriving on the contradictions. Typical approaches would include combining or integrating apparently opposing interpretations or solutions rather than choosing or arguing for one interpretation/solution over its opposite. Such approaches are more likely to lead to effective performance in the constantly changing situations work where contradictions are common or even inherently present. Those who are less tolerant of contradictions (but similarly high on SJA), on the other hand, would attempt to remove the contradiction by actively seeking out information or behaving in ways that would hopefully rule out one interpretation or solution in favor of its opposite. Their high SJA would provide them the cognitive and motivational basis to generate, with great conviction, strong arguments for one of the two opposing positions and strong counter-arguments to the other. However, given the many contradictions present in work situations, attempts at removing most of them are likely to be unsuccessful or even maladaptive and lead to ineffective performance. The constant arguments and counter-arguments would lead to disagreements with others (coworkers, supervisors) who hold the opposing position. In short, among individuals who are similarly high on SJA, job performance should increase as TC increases.

The converse is probably true for individuals low on SJA. That is, the tendency to tolerate contradictions in a work situation is likely to be maladaptive in terms of job performance when the individual is low on SJA. This is because individuals low on SJA are less likely to be able to correctly recognize the relevant dynamic situational features and separate them from unimportant details or nondynamic features. Hence, they are more ignorant or less appreciative of the actual presence and absence of apparent contradictions. Among these individuals, those who are more tolerant of contradictions would accept all seemingly contradictory positions at face value, regardless whether or not one of the opposing positions is in fact invalid or inferior, or even when the contradictions are not real. They would mistakenly (due to their low SJA) combine these opposing positions to arrive at a suboptimal or maladaptive judgment, decision, or response thereby leading to ineffective performance, as compared to those who are low in TC who would not combine opposing positions. In contrast, those who are less tolerant of contradictions would attempt to remove the contradiction by actions such as seeking additional information to rule out one of the opposing positions. They are more likely to perform better than those who are more TC (who mistakenly combined the positions) because there is at least a chance for them to correctly rule out the inferior or invalid position. Unlike those who are low on TC but high on SJA, these individuals are less likely to produce strong arguments or counter-arguments with much conviction due to their lower SJA. Their relatively weaker arguments and counter-arguments are less likely to lead to disagreements with others (coworkers, supervisors) who hold the opposing position. In fact, they may also reconcile the contradiction simply by adopting the position of others instead of their initial position. However, they will tend not to perform as well as those who are high on both TC and SJA who are able to accurately identify inherent contradictions and respond effectively by integrating the contradictory positions. Based on the aforementioned conceptualizations of the joint effects of TC and SJA, it is predicted that:

H2:   Situational Judgment Ability (SJA) and Tolerance for Contradiction
(TC) will have a crossover disordinal interaction effect on job perfor-

mance such that TC and job performance are positively associated when SJA is high but negatively associated when SJA is low.

In addition, all the aforementioned specific conceptualizations will be supported if the interaction predicted in H2 shows the following pattern: (a) the level of job performance will be highest for individuals who are high on both SJA and TC and lowest for those who are high on SJA but low on TC as well as those who are high on TC but low on SJA, (b) there will be no difference in performance level between those who are high on SJA but low on TC and those who are high on TC but low on SJA, and (c) those who are low on both SJA and TC will have a moderate level of job performance that is lower than those who are high on SJA and high on TC but higher than those who are high on SJA but low on TC as well as those who are high on TC but low on SJA.

Method

Participants and procedure.   A total of 142 prison officers (24% women) from the Singapore Prison Service voluntarily completed the measures as part of a larger study (unpublished) on test validation. The sample has a mean organizational tenure of 7.93 years (SD = 3.53) and a mean age of 30.80 years (SD = 3.97). Participants completed all measures in groups of about 20 in classroom settings. They were told that the purpose of this study was to examine problem-solving styles. All participants were debriefed.

Measures.   SJA was assessed using a situational judgment test that was developed by the author as part of the larger test validation study for the Singapore Prison Service. The procedure for developing the test and the test format were similar to that reported in Chan and Schmitt (2002) but the test content was different. The test content was specifically designed to measure prison officers' overall ability to make judgments in and respond effectively to practical work-related situations that may arise in a variety of jobs similar to those in the Prison Service. Using task statements and work-related competencies generated in a job analysis of the prison officer positions, the author discussed facets of situational judgment with two groups of subject matter experts (n_1 = 12, n_2 = 15) who had been in supervisory positions for 4 to 10 years. The final form of the situational judgment test was obtained after a series of test revisions based on discussions with another group of five subject matter experts and three psychology graduate students. The final test consisted of eight situations with 40 items (i.e., 5 items per situation). Five alternative responses (i.e., items) were presented to the examinee following the description of each situation. Examinees' scores on the test were computed on the basis of their endorsement of the effectiveness of the responses using a six-point Likert-type rating scale with anchors ranging from 1 (*very ineffective*) to 6 (*very effective*). The scoring key was developed from prior effectiveness ratings of response alternatives obtained from on-the-job subject matter experts. Using percentage of agreement among subject matter expert, participants' effectiveness rating on each of the 40 items received a score of 0, 1, or 2, with higher scores representing higher SJA. Principal component analyses performed on the situational judgment responses on the 40 items indicated that a single-factor solution provided a reasonable fit to the data accounting for 22% of the variance. Consistent with previous research on situational judgment tests, no multiple interpretable factors were identified. Thus, it was most meaningful to use a single total test score in our analyses to represent SJA. The Cronbach's alpha estimate of internal consistency reliability was only .74 for the relatively long test (i.e., 40 items), which is typical of situational judgment tests. Similar relatively low internal consistency reliabilities for a 40-item test (.73) and a 33-item test (.45 to .74 across three groups) were reported by Chan and Schmitt (2002) and Pulakos and Schmitt (1996), respectively.

Tolerance for Contradiction was assessed with the same 10-item TCS used in Study 1. *Job Performance* was measured using supervisory ratings obtained as part of Study 2; all participants were rated by their supervisors on a 3-item measure using a 5-point Likert-type rating scale ranging from 1 (*strongly disagree*) to 5 (*strongly agree*). The items were "This officer's overall work quality is high," "This officer is good at meeting performance standards," and "This officer is competent in performing his/her job tasks." Cronbach's alpha of the measure was .82.

Data analyses.   Principal component analyses and confirmatory factor analyses (including multiple-group analyses) were used to test the one-factor structure of the TCS. In addition, multiple-group confirmatory factor analyses were used to test for measurement invariance of responses between the prison officer sample in Study 2 and the undergraduate sample in Study 1. This was accomplished by fitting a series of three nested multiple-group models that differ on whether factor loadings and error variances were freely estimated or constrained to be equal across the two groups (i.e., samples). In all three models (all models specified a one-factor structure), the factor variance was freely estimated across the two groups. For all three models, Item 1 on the measure was used in both groups as the reference indicator with factor loading fixed to 1.00 for scaling purpose. Equality of factor loadings would provide evidence of measurement invariance between groups. Even stronger evidence of measurement invariance would be provided if there were equality of both factor loadings and error variances between groups, although the strict criterion of equality of error variances is typically not necessary as a condition for measurement invariance (Alwin & Jackson, 1981; MacCallum & Tucker, 1991). Correlational and hierarchical regression analyses were used to test the SJA–job performance relation and the SJA × TC interaction effect on job performance predicted in H1 and H2, respectively.

Results and Discussion

Principal component analysis performed on the 10 TCS items clearly indicated a single factor solution, as indicated by the scree plot. The single dominant factor accounted for 45% of the total variance, which was comparable to the proportion of variance accounted for in Study 1 (i.e., 40%). The confirmatory factor analysis showed that a single factor model provided a good fit to the data, as indicated by a convergence of good fit from the various established model fit indexes (NNFI = .97, CFI = .98, SRMR = .05, RMSEA = .06). All standardized factor loadings were significant ($p < .05$) and of substantial magnitude ranging from .32 to .56 with a mean loading of .42. To test for measurement invariance between the prison officer sample in Study 2 and the undergraduate sample in Study 1, a series of three nested multiple-group confirmatory factor analytic models were fitted to the two 10×10 item variance–covariance matrices. As shown in Table 3, the nested model comparison between M1 and M2 showed no significant between-groups (samples) differences in factor loadings ($\Delta\chi^2 = 10$, $\Delta df = 9$, $p > .05$). Moreover, the practical fit indexes remained virtually identical from M1 to M2. Hence, there was evidence of measurement invariance of responses between the two study groups. However, the stricter criterion that requires equality of error variances between groups was not fulfilled, as indicated by the significant chi square difference between models M2

TABLE 3
Fit Indexes Associated With Multiple-Group Confirmatory Factor Analytic
Models for Tests of Measurement Invariance of Responses Between
Undergraduates[a] and Prison Officers[b]

Model Comparison	df	χ^2	Model Comparison	Δdf	$\Delta\chi^2$	NNFI	CFI	SRMR	RMSEA
M1: Free factor loadings; free error variances	70	151*				.95	.96	.05	.08
M2: Equal factor loadings; free error variances	79	161*	M1 vs. M2	9	10	.95	.96	.06	.08
M3: Equal factor loadings; equal error variances	89	420*	M2 vs. M3	10	259*	.82	.83	.14	.14

Note. All three multiple-group models specified a single factor for the undergraduate group and the prison officer group. In all three models, factor variance was freely estimated across the two groups. For all three models, Item 1 on the measure was used in both groups as the reference indicator with factor loading fixed to 1.00 for scaling purpose. Model M2 was selected as the most adequate (based on model fit indices and parsimony) representation of the data. NNFI = nonnormed fit index; CFI = Comparative Fit Index; SRMR = standardized root mean square residual; RMSEA = root mean square error of approximation.

[a]Study 1, $N = 198$. [b]Study 2, $N = 142$.

*$p < .05$.

and M3 ($\Delta\chi^2 = 259$, $\Delta df = 10$, $p < .05$). Moreover, M3 did not provide a good fit to the data, as indicated by the practical model fit indexes. Hence, the constrained model (M2) that specified equality of corresponding factor loadings across the two groups was selected as the most adequate (based on model fit and parsimony) model for representing the data. The Cronbach's alpha for the TCS in Study 2 was .86, which was acceptable and similar in magnitude to that obtained in Study 1 (i.e., .83). In summary, similar to Study 1, Study 2 obtained substantial evidence that the TCS was unitary. In addition, measurement invariance of responses was established between the prison officer sample in Study 2 and the undergraduate sample in Study 1, providing evidence that the 10 items on the TCS function similarly across the two studies.

The descriptive statistics of the study variables are presented in Table 4. As expected, TC was uncorrelated with SJA ($r = .01$, $p > .05$). This empirical null association is consistent with the conceptual distinction between the two variables, a distinction that was assumed in the arguments for H1 and H2.

H1 predicted that SJA will positively predict job performance but that there will be no association between TC and job performance. As shown in Table 4, SJA was significantly and positively correlated with job performance ($r = .28$, $p < .05$) whereas TC was uncorrelated with job performance ($r = .03$, $p > .05$). Hence, H1 was supported. This pattern of correlations with job performance provided further convergent evidence that tolerance for contradiction and SJA are distinct constructs.

H2 predicted that a SJA × TC crossover disordinal interaction effect on job performance such that TC and job performance are positively associated when SJA is high but negatively associated when SJA is low. Table 5 summarizes the hierarchical regression analyses performed to test the interaction. As shown in the table, SJA and TC were entered as a single block in Step 1 of the regression of job performance. The two variables jointly accounted for a significant 8% ($p < .05$) of the job performance variance, but with virtually all the variance accounted for provided by SJA ($\beta = .28$, $p < .05$) and none from TC ($\beta = .03$, $p > .05$). This is consistent with the pattern of zero-order correlations reported in Table 4. The SJA × TC interaction

TABLE 4
Means, Standard Deviations, Reliabilities, and Correlations of
Study 2 Variables

Variable	M	SD	1	2	3
1. Tolerance for contradiction	3.76	.45	(.86)		
2. Situational judgment ability	57.60	16.95	.01	(.74)	
3. Job performance	4.28	.55	.03	.28*	(.82)

Note. $N = 142$. Values in parentheses represent reliabilities obtained in this study.
*$p < .05$.

TABLE 5
Summary of Hierarchical Regression Analyses for Test of SJA × TC
Interaction Effect on Job Performance

Variable	β	R^2	df	ΔR^2	Δdf
Step 1					
SJA	0.28*	.08*	2		
TC	0.03				
Step 2					
SJA × TC	3.81*	.21*	3	.13*	1

Note. $N = 142$. SJA = Situational Judgment Ability; TC = Tolerance for Contradiction; β = the standardized regression coefficients associated with each step of the regression.
    *$p < .05$.

term was then entered in Step 2 of the regression. Entering this interaction term resulted in a significant 13% increase in variance accounted for, $p < .05$. To understand the nature of this interaction effect, the interaction was plotted using established procedure described in Aiken and West (1991). As shown in Figure 1, the SJA × TC interaction was of the same crossover disordinal nature as hypothesized in H2. Specifically, TC and job performance are positively associated when SJA is high but negatively associated when SJA is low. Hence, H2 was supported.

To elaborate on the finding of the crossover interaction in H2, Cohen's *d* was computed for the relevant pairs of points corresponding to high (+1 SD) and low

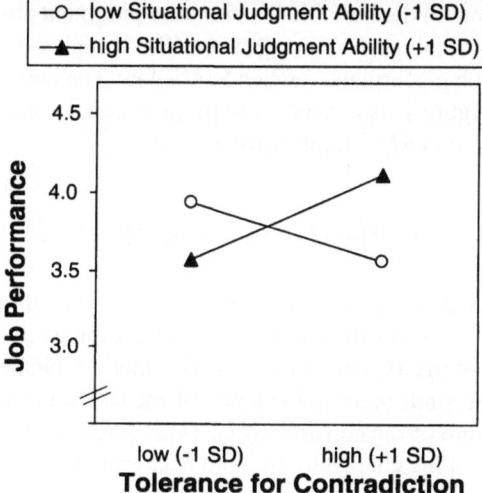

FIGURE 1   Interaction of situational judgment ability and tolerance for contradiction on job performance.

(–1 SD) levels of SJA and TC. As shown in Figure 1, the level of job performance was highest for individuals who are high on both SJA (+1 SD) and TC (+1 SD) and lowest for those who are high on SJA (+1 SD) but low on TC (–1 SD) as well as those who are high on TC (+1 SD) but low on SJA (–1 SD). The difference in performance levels were significant ($p < .05$) and large with a magnitude of one standard deviation unit, between "high SJA and high TC" and "high SJA & low TC" ($d = .98$) and between "high SJA and high TC" and "high TC and low SJA" ($d = 1.00$). There was no significant difference in performance levels between "high SJA and low TC" and "high TC and low SJA" ($d = .02, p > .05$). Those who are low on both SJA and TC had a moderate level of job performance that was significantly ($p < .05$) lower than "high SJA and high TC" ($d = .31$) but higher than "high SJA and low TC" ($d = .67$) and "high TC & low SJA" ($d = .69$). Among individuals with a moderate level of SJA (mean), there was no significant difference in performance level between those who are high on TC and those who are low on TC ($d = .14, p > .05$). This is consistent with the overall null association between TC and job performance as reported earlier (i.e., part of H1).

In summary, Study 2 found additional evidence for the TCS as a measure of the TC construct. The unidimensional factor structure of the measure and its reliability obtained in Study 1 with the undergraduate sample were replicated in Study 2 with the prison officer sample. In addition, the measure has demonstrated measurement invariance across the two samples that have very different demographic profiles and background characteristics. TC has been shown to be distinct from SJA. Although the construct has no overall association ("main effect") on job performance, TC is relevant to job performance because it may be either adaptive or maladaptive depending on the individual's situation judgment ability. TC is adaptive (positively predicts job performance) when SJA is high but it is maladaptive (negatively predicts job performance) when SJA is low. The pattern of the interaction, as depicted in Figure 1, is consistent with the specific conceptualizations of the joint effects of TC and SJA on job performance.

GENERAL DISCUSSION

These results provide preliminary evidence for individual differences in TC in three different ways. First, results from both studies support the convergent and discriminant validity of the TC construct vis-à-vis other established individual difference constructs. Second, there is evidence of measurement invariance of the unidimensional measure of the construct (i.e., TCS) across two disparate samples with different demographic characteristics and background characteristics. Third, TC is relevant to the workplace and is important, both conceptually and practically, because it can have either adaptive or maladaptive consequences in that it can either positively or negatively predict job performance depending on the individual's

level of SJA. TC has a positive impact on job performance when SJA is high but a negative impact when SJA is low.

Although the evidence from the two studies reported here is promising, it is premature to specify precise practical implications for work psychology (e.g., personnel selection) at this time without further research, given several limitations in the present two studies. First, both studies did not have the opportunity to collect repeated-measures data to compute test–retest reliability or other stability coefficients that will provide stronger evidence for TC as a true individual difference construct as opposed to a readily malleable problem-solving style. Second, the extent to which the findings will cross-validate in a wider variety of samples remains unknown. In particular, research using different samples and job contexts is needed to test the robustness of the SJA × TC interaction found in Study 2. Third, future studies are needed to identify the boundary conditions for the relations obtained in the two studies outlined in this article, especially Study 2. For example, job type, job level, and specific organizational climates are possible boundary conditions for the influence of individual differences in TC on job-relevant criteria. Fourth, the type of criterion is likely to determine the nature of the TC–criterion relation. Hence, future construct validation efforts need to be guided by the nature of the criterion and the specification of the type of "fuzzy demands" or demands on reasoning about contradictions that exist in the situation of interest. A potentially fruitful research in this direction is to examine the effects of the degree of fit or misfit between individuals' level of TC and the type of situational demands. This may be investigated at the level of person–job, person–group, person–organization, or even person–culture fit/misfit. It would be interesting to examine if and when the effects of fit and misfit are asymmetrical. Finally, other individual difference constructs or situational variables may also interact with TC to affect important criterion outcomes. To prevent the accumulation of "positive" findings obtained through capitalization on chance, our search for these interacting variables should be theory-driven. We should adopt a construct-oriented approach that relates TC to the conceptual definitions of the individual difference or situational variables that are potential interacting variables.

This is the first attempt in the literature to conceptualize, measure, and validate TC as an *individual difference* construct where individuals may be located on a *quantitative* continuum ranging from low to high TC. A strict bivalent thinker and a strict fuzzy thinker are simply ideal types on the bipolar ends of this quantitative continuum. The approach adopted here differs in several substantive ways from the recent stream of research on cultural differences in reasoning by Nisbett and colleagues (Nisbett, 2003; Nisbett, Peng, Choi, & Norenzayan, 2001; Peng & Nisbett, 1999). First, Nisbett and colleagues treat differences in reasoning about contradictions as a *qualitative* difference in thought processes between cultures. According to these authors, the process of thinking and reasoning about contradictions is qualitatively (not quantitatively) different between Chinese cultures and European

American cultures and the difference is rooted in the different naïve metaphysical systems and tacit epistemologies in the two cultures (Nisbett et al., 2001). Nisbett et al. argued that the responses to thinking or reasoning tasks are qualitatively different between Chinese (or East Asians) and European Americans (or Westerners) and that "these qualitative differences indicate that literally different cognitive processes are often invoked by East Asians and Westerners dealing with the same problem" (p. 305).

Nisbett and colleagues argued that the Chinese are dialectical thinkers who embrace change, holism, and contradictions whereas European American thinkers are nondialectical and analytical thinkers who adhere to logical principles equivalent to Aristotle's laws of bivalent logic. Because dialectical thinking is construed as holistic cognition that is unique to the Chinese system of thought and qualitatively different from the analytical cognition in the European American system of thought, within-Chinese culture differences in dialectical thinking and within-European American differences in analytical thinking are statistically construed as error variance in the empirical research by Nisbett and colleagues, although it is less clear if within-culture individual differences can also be treated as a theoretical construct in its own right. This contrasts with the present conceptualization of TC that explicitly treats (within-culture) individual differences on the variable as true construct variance. The present conceptualization does not rule out between-culture mean differences in TC but the mean differences would be treated as quantitative differences that are not conceptually (i.e., qualitatively) distinct from mean differences between any subgroups within the same culture. The treatment of between-culture differences (as quantitative or qualitative difference) is critical because it affects the legitimacy of the direct comparisons of scores on the same measurement scale. Direct comparison of absolute differences (alpha change) between cultures (or other groups) is not meaningful if there are in fact qualitative differences in the measurement responses due to differences in subjective calibration of the scale (beta change) or conceptualization of the construct (gamma change; see Chan, 1998a; Drasgow, 1984; Golembiewski, Billingsley, & Yeager, 1976; Millsap & Hartog, 1988).

A second difference between the present work and the research by Nisbett and colleagues is that TC, as conceptualized here, is only one of three facets of dialectical thinking and therefore conceptually less complex than dialectical thinking. The author is currently developing and validating measures of individual differences in the other two facets of dialectical thinking, namely, *change* and *holism*. Having individual difference measures of all three facets of dialectical thinking would allow the empirical assessments of interfacet comparisons, interfacet relations, as well as the validity of alternative factorial structures of the composite. This would in turn provide a more commensurable basis to compare the individual-level constructs and the construct of dialectical thinking that is at the culture level. It remains an empirical question to be answered in future research on whether dialectical thinking is better conceptualized as an irreducible culture construct or a group-level construct that is composed from the TC construct conceptualized and measured at the individual level of analysis. To establish a group-level construct from an individual-level construct, we would need to identify and test an appropriate *composition model* (Chan, 1998b) that specifies the functional relations between the similar constructs at the different levels of analysis. Whether or not the two conceptualizations (i.e., irreducible culture construct versus composed group-level construct) are consistent will depend on the specific type of composition model specified.

In conclusion, this article offers promising but preliminary evidence that individuals differ in TC and that these differences can be measured with psychometric validity. More construct validation research is needed. Given the potential importance of the construct, more research on individual differences in TC appears warranted.

REFERENCES

Aiken, L. S., & West, S. G. (1991). *Multiple regression: Testing and interpreting interactions.* Newbury Park, CA: Sage.

Alwin, D. F., & Jackson, D. J. (1981). Applications of simultaneous factor analysis to issues of factorial invariance. In D. Jackson & E. Borgatta (Eds.), *Factor analysis and measurement in sociological research: A multidimensional perspective* (pp. 249–279). Beverly Hills, CA: Sage.

Ashford, S. J., & Cummings, L. L. (1985). Proactive feedback seeking: The instrumental use of the information environment. *Journal of Occupational Psychology, 58,* 67–97.

Bateman, T. S., & Crant, J. M. (1993). The proactive component of organizational behavior: A measure and correlates. *Journal of Organizational Behavior, 14,* 103–118.

Chan, D. (1996). Cognitive misfit of problem-solving style at work: A facet of person–organization fit. *Organizational Behavior and Human Decision Processes, 68,* 194–207.

Chan, D. (1998a). The conceptualization and analysis of change over time: An integrative approach incorporating longitudinal means and covariance structures analysis (LMACS) and multiple indicator latent growth modeling (MLGM). *Organizational Research Methods, 1,* 421–483.

Chan, D. (1998b). Functional relations among constructs in the same content domain at different levels of analysis: A typology of composition models. *Journal of Applied Psychology, 83,* 234–246.

Chan, D. (2000). Understanding adaptation to changes in the work environment: Integrating individual difference and learning perspectives. *Research in Personnel and Human Resources Management, 18,* 1–42.

Chan, D. (2001). Method effects of positive affectivity, negative affectivity, and impression management in self-reports of work attitudes. *Human Performance, 14,* 77–96.

Chan, D., & Schmitt, N. (2002). Situational judgment and job performance. *Human Performance, 15,* 233–254.

Chan, D., & Sim, C. (2002, April). *Individual differences in fuzzy thinking.* Paper presented at the 17th Annual Conference of the Society for Industrial and Organizational Psychology, Toronto, Canada.

Cheeseman, P. (1986). Probabilistic versus fuzzy reasoning. In L. N. Kanal & J. F. Lemmer (Eds.), *Uncertainty in artificial intelligence* (pp. 85–102). New York: Elsevier.

Clevenger, J., Pereira, G. M., Wiechmann, D., Schmitt, N., & Harvey, V. S. (2001). Incremental validity of situational judgment tests. *Journal of Applied Psychology, 86,* 410–417.

Costa, P. T., Jr., & McCrae, R., R. (1992). *NEO PI-R: Professional manual. Revised NEO Personality Inventory (NEO-PI-R) and NEO Five-Factor Inventory (NEO-FFI).* Odessa, FL: Psychological Assessment Resources.

Crant, J. M. (1995). The proactive personality scale and objective job performance among real estate agents. *Journal of Applied Psychology, 80,* 532–537.

Crant, J. M. (1996). The proactive personality scale as a predictor of entrepreneurial intentions. *Journal of Small Business Management, 34*(3), 42–49.

Crant, J. M., & Bateman, T. S. (2000). Charismatic leadership viewed from above: The impact of proactive personality. *Journal of Organizational Behavior, 21,* 63–75.

Digman, M. J. (1990). Personality structure: Emergence of the five-factor model. *Annual Review of Psychology, 41,* 417–440.

Drasgow, F. (1984). Scrutinizing psychological tests: Measurement equivalence and equivalent relations with external variables are central issues. *Psychological Bulletin, 95,* 134–135.

Dubios, D., Nguyen, H. T., Prade, H., & Segeno, M. (1999). Introduction: The real contribution of fuzzy systems. In H. T. Nguyen & M. Segeno (Eds.), *Fuzzy systems: Modeling and control* (pp. 1–17). Netherlands: Kluwer.

Furnham, A. (1994). A content, correlational and factor analytic study of four tolerance of ambiguity questionnaires. *Personality and Individual Differences, 16,* 403–410.

Golembiewski, R. T., Billingsley, K., & Yeager, S. (1976). Measuring change and persistence in human affairs: Types of change generated by OD designs. *Journal of Applied Behavioral Science, 12,* 133–157.

Jonassen, H. D., & Grabowski, B. L. (1993). *Handbook of individual differences, learning, and instruction.* Hillsdale, NJ: Lawrence Erlbaum Associates, Inc.

Kirkman, B. L., & Rosen, B. (1999). Beyond self-management: Antecedents and consequences of team empowerment. *Academy of Management Journal, 42,* 58–74.

Kosko, B. (1993). *Tolerance for contradiction: The new science of fuzzy logic.* New York: Hyperion.

MacCallum, R. C., & Tucker, L. R. (1991). Representing sources of error in the common-factor model: Implications for theory and practice. *Psychological Bulletin, 109,* 502–511.

Massaro, D. W., & Cohen, M. M. (1993). The paradigm and the fuzzy logical model of perception are alive and well. *Journal of Experimental Psychology: General, 122,* 115–124.

McDaniel, M. A., Morgeson, F. P., Finnegan, E. B., Campion, M. A., & Braverman, E. P. (2001). Predicting job performance using situational judgment tests: A clarification of the literature. *Journal of Applied Psychology, 86,* 730–740.

McNeill, D., & Freiberger, P. (1993). *Fuzzy logic.* New York: Simon & Schuster.

Millsap, R. E., & Hartog, S. B. (1988). Alpha, beta, and gamma change in evaluation research: A structural equation approach. *Journal of Applied Psychology, 73,* 574–584.

Mount, M. K., & Barrick, M. R. (1998). Five reasons why the "Big Five" article had been frequently cited. *Personnel Psychology, 51,* 848–857.

Neuberg, L. S., & Newsom, T. J. (1993). Personal need for structure: Individual differences in the desire for simple structure. *Journal of Personality and Social Psychology, 65*(1), 113–131.

Nisbett, R. E. (2003). *The geography of thought: How Asians and Westerners think differently and why.* London: Nicholas Brealey.

Nisbett, R. E., Peng, K., Choi, I., & Norenzayan, A. (2001). Culture and systems of thought: Holistic versus analytic cognition. *Psychological Review, 108,* 291–310.

Norton, R. (1975). Measurement of ambiguity tolerance. *Journal of Personality Assessment, 39,* 607–619.

Pal, S. K. (1991). Fuzzy tools for the management of uncertainty in pattern recognition, image analysis, vision, and expert systems. *International Journal of Systems Science, 22,* 511–549.

Parker, S. K., & Sprigg, C. A. (1999). Minimizing strain and maximizing learning: The role of job demands, job control, and proactive personality. *Journal of Applied Psychology, 84,* 925–939.

Paulhus, D. L. (1984). Two components models of socially desirable responding. *Journal of Personality and Social Psychology, 46*, 598–609.

Paulhus, D. L. (1988). *Assessing self-deception and impression management in self-reports: The Balanced Inventory of Desirable Responding.* Unpublished manual, University of British Columbia, Vancouver, Canada.

Peng, K., & Nisbett, R. E. (1999). Culture, dialectics, and reasoning about contradiction. *American Psychologist, 54*, 741–754.

Pulakos, E. D., Arad, S., Donovan, M. A., & Plamondon, K. E. (2000). Adaptability in the workplace: Development of a taxonomy of adaptive performance. *Journal of Applied Psychology, 85*, 612–624.

Pulakos, E. D., & Schmitt, N. (1996). An evaluation of two strategies for reducing adverse impact and their effects on criterion-related validity. *Human Performance, 9*, 241–258.

Rasiowa, H. (1993). Toward fuzzy logic. In L. A. Zadeh & J. Kacprzyk (Eds.), *Fuzzy logic for the management of uncertainty* (pp. 7–11). New York: Wiley.

Rayner, S., & Riding, R. (1997). Towards a categorization of cognitive styles and learning styles. *Educational Psychology, 17*, 5–27.

Reyna, V. F., & Brainerd, C. J. (1992). Fuzzy trace theory on reasoning and remembering: Paradoxes, patterns, and parallelism. In A. F. Healy, S. M. Kosslyn, & R. M. Shiffrin (Eds.), *From learning processes to cognitive processes: Essays in honor of William K. Estes* (Vol. 2, pp. 235–259). Hillsdale, NJ: Lawrence Erlbaum Associates, Inc.

Seibert, S. E., Crant, J. M., & Kraimer, M. L. (1999). Proactive personality and career success. *Journal of Applied Psychology, 84*, 416–427.

Sternberg, R. J. (1997). *Thinking styles.* Cambridge University Press.

Sternberg, R. J., Wagner, R. W., & Okagaki, L. (1993). Practical intelligence: The nature and role of tacit knowledge at work and school. In H. Reese & J. Puckett (Eds.), *Advances in lifespan development* (pp. 195–227). Hillsdale, NJ: Lawrence Erlbaum Associates, Inc.

Tucker, P., & Warr, P. (1996). Intelligence, elementary cognitive components, and cognitive styles as predictors of complex task performance. *Personality and Individual Differences, 21*(1), 91–102.

Viswanathan, M. (1997). Individual differences in need for precision. *Personality and Social Psychology Bulletin, 23*, 717–735.

Wagner, R. K., & Sternberg, R. J. (1985). Practical intelligence in real world pursuits: The role of tacit knowledge. *Journal of Personality and Social Psychology, 48*, 436–458.

Watson, D., Clark, A. L., & Tellegen, A. (1988). Development and validation of brief measures of positive and negative affect: The PANAS scales. *Journal of Personality and Social Psychology, 54*, 1063–1070.

Zadeh, L. (1965). Fuzzy sets. *Information and Control, 8*, 338–353.

Zadeh, L. (1980). Fuzzy sets versus probability. *Proceedings of the IEEE, 68*, 421.

APPENDIX
The Tolerance for Contradiction Scale (TCS)

Instructions

This questionnaire is designed for you to indicate the typical ways in which you approach or solve problems in everyday life. There are no right or wrong answers. For each item, please use the following 5-point rating scale to indicate the extent to which you agree or disagree that the statement accurately describes the way you

typically approach or solve problems. Write the appropriate number on the line
___ provided at the end of each statement.

1 = strongly disagree
2 = disagree
3 = neutral; neither disagree nor agree
4 = agree
5 = strongly agree

---

1. When a problem appears to have two equally effective but opposing solutions, it is likely that the problem has been poorly defined or poorly represented. ___*
2. When faced with a puzzling issue in which there are two opposing but equally possible interpretations, I would typically gather information to rule out one of the two interpretations.___ *
3. When my friend's view on an issue is opposite to my view, I usually think of situations in which both my view and my friend's view can be valid at the same time. ___
4. People who often give ambiguous answers when answering a question should take a position and give a more exact answer. ___*
5. People who maintain that it is possible for two opposing interpretations of the same event to be both true are illogical or unrealistic. ___*
6. Within a team, cooperation and competition can exist at the same time. ___
7. A single action or behavior can often achieve opposite objectives at the same time. ___
8. "If A is true, then B must be true. If B is false, then C must be true. Given that A is false, is C true or false?" Such questions lead to ineffective problem-solving skills in many areas of life. ___
9. In assessing whether someone is supporting a team, team members often make statements such as "He is either for us or against us." Team members who make such statements fail to see many other real possibilities. ___
10. In most situations, whether an act is morally right or wrong is clear cut. ___*

---

* = reverse-scored. The mean of the 10 items is used to represent Tolerance for Contradiction, with higher values representing higher levels on the construct.

HUMAN PERFORMANCE, *17*(3), 325–346

Emotional Stability, Core Self-Evaluations, and Job Outcomes: A Review of the Evidence and an Agenda for Future Research

Timothy A. Judge
Warrington College of Business
University of Florida

Annelies E. M. Van Vianen and Irene E. De Pater
Department of Work and Organizational Psychology
University of Amsterdam

In this article we present a review of research on core self-evaluations, a broad personality trait indicated by 4 more narrow traits: self-esteem, generalized self-efficacy, locus of control, and emotional stability. We review evidence suggesting that the 4 core traits are highly related, load on a single unitary factor, and have dubious incremental validity controlling for their common core. We more generally investigate the construct validity of core self-evaluations. We also report on the development and validation of the first direct measure of the concept, the Core Self-Evaluations Scale (CSES). Cross-cultural evidence on the CSES is provided. We conclude by offering an agenda for future research, discussing areas where future core self-evaluations research is most needed.

Emotional stability or neuroticism is perhaps the most enduring personality concept in psychology. There are thousands of studies on the topic and the entire field of psychoanalysis and clinical psychology might be traced to the study of neurotic symptoms (Freud, 1910). In the realm of normal psychology, the findings regarding the importance of neuroticism to applied criteria, such as job performance and

---

Requests for reprints should be sent to Timothy A. Judge, Department of Management, 211D Stuzin Hall, Warrington College of Business, University of Florida, Gainesville, FL 32611. E-mail: timothy.judge@cba.ufl.edu

job satisfaction, are somewhat contradictory. There are several meta-analyses of the relation of neuroticism to job performance. The first two of these analyses were published nearly concurrently but found substantially different results. In their meta-analysis, Barrick and Mount (1991) found that the relation between emotional stability and job performance was not significantly different from zero ($\rho = .08$) across criterion measures. Tett, Jackson, and Rothstein (1991), using different inclusion criteria but flawed analytical procedures, found a corrected mean correlation of $-.22$ between neuroticism and job performance. Recently, in a third meta-analysis, using a European Community sample, Salgado (1997) estimated a true validity of .19 for emotional stability. As a part of a larger study, Judge and Bono (2001a) recently conducted yet another meta-analysis of neuroticism and job performance, using only direct measures of neuroticism. Results of this study produced the same validity estimate as Salgado, $\rho = .19$. Although explanation of these conflicting findings has been offered with respect to the first two studies (Ones, Mount, Barrick, & Hunter, 1994) and there has been an effort to integrate prior meta-analyses (Barrick, Mount, & Judge, 2001), the nature of the relation of emotional stability to job performance remains uncertain.

The relation between neuroticism and job satisfaction has also been examined, providing perhaps more consistent evidence. Several studies have shown that direct measures of neuroticism are negatively related to job satisfaction (Furnham & Zacherl, 1986; Smith, Organ, & Near, 1983; Tokar & Subich, 1997). Judge and Bono's (2001a) recent meta-analysis revealed a correlation of $\rho = .24$ between emotional stability and job satisfaction. Though this correlation was distinguishable from zero, it may be surprising that the correlation was not stronger.

It is possible that the contradictory findings regarding the relation of emotional stability to job performance and, to a lesser extent, job satisfaction, are due to the measurement of emotional stability. Specifically, it is possible that typical measures of emotional stability do not adequately measure the broad concept, and do so to varying degrees, such that one observes validities that are both lower and more variable than one would observe with broader measures that better indicate the concept. One suggestion for how emotional stability might be more broadly measured was provided by Judge, Locke, and Durham (1997) in the form of core self-evaluations. Accordingly, the purpose of this article is to discuss the concept of core self-evaluations and note how this concept, as a broad measure of emotional stability, may lead to higher and more consistent validities.

CORE SELF-EVALUATIONS: NATURE
OF THE CONSTRUCT

Core self-evaluations is a higher order concept representing the fundamental evaluations that people make about themselves and their functioning in their environment. Individuals with positive core self-evaluations appraise themselves in a consistently positive manner across situations; such individuals see themselves as capable, worthy, and in control of their lives. According to Judge et al. (1997), the core self-evaluations concept is indicated by four traits: self-esteem, locus of control, neuroticism, and generalized self-efficacy. Judge, Bono, Erez, Locke, and Thoresen (2002) presented evidence that the first three of these traits are the most widely studied in psychology. Curiously, however, the quest to find broad personality factors has ignored the commonality among these traits. Although neuroticism has been considered a broad trait even by those researchers who do not endorse the five-factor model (Eysenck, 1990), self-esteem and locus of control continue to be studied as individual, isolated traits. We argue that consideration of these traits in isolation leads to underprediction and semantic confusion (Dewey, 1974).

Conceptually, the traits share many similarities. For example, all of the core traits assess the positivity of self-description. Similarly, it appears that individuals who score low on each of the core traits are more susceptible to self-relevant social cues (e.g., Brockner, 1979; Hjelle & Clouser, 1970). There are a few studies that have investigated the relation among other pairs of the core traits (e.g., self-esteem and locus of control, Francis, 1996; locus of control and neuroticism, Morrison, 1997), though none of these studies explicitly consider the possibility that these traits may indicate a common higher order concept. That the individual core traits may share conceptual and empirical similarities does not demonstrate, however, that core self-evaluations is a valid psychological construct. To do that, one must analyze core self-evaluations from a construct validity perspective. In the next section of this article, we provide a detailed analysis of the construct validity of the core self-evaluations concept.

CONSTRUCT VALIDITY OF CORE SELF-EVALUATIONS

As Schwab (1980) argued, establishing the validity of a psychological concept involves both conceptual issues (definition and theoretical relations with other variables) and empirical considerations (convergent validity and location of the concept within its nomological network). In ascertaining the validity of the core self-evaluations concept, four issues must be addressed:

1. *Convergent validity.* To demonstrate convergent validity, the four core self-evaluations traits (self-esteem, locus of control, neuroticism, and generalized self-efficacy) must share sufficient covariance to indicate a common concept.
2. *Lack of discriminant validity of core traits.* If the core traits fail to display differential patterns of relations with other variables, then the core traits would lack discriminant validity relative to one another. This would further support the argument that the four core traits indicate a common construct.

3. *Discriminant validity relative to other traits.* To be useful, the core concept must be distinct from other traits, such as the traits from the five-factor model of personality (excluding emotional stability, of course).

4. *Predictive validity.* Predictive validity is revealed by the degree to which the core factor predicts criteria better than the isolated core traits or beyond other traits (such as the Big Five traits).

Convergent Validity

Convergent validity refers to whether measures show sufficient interrelations to demonstrate that they indicate the same concept. In terms of core self-evaluations theory, the question of convergent validity can be answered by examining the correlations among the four core traits. Table 1 provides the correlations among the core self-evaluations traits based on meta-analytic data reported in Judge, Erez, Bono, and Thoresen (2002). As the table shows, the correlations are substantial. The average correlation among the traits (.64) is at least as high as the correlations among alternative measures of traits in the five-factor model (see Ones, 1993). Another piece of evidence in favor of the core concept is factor analytic research that consistently suggests the four core traits load on a common factor, both in confirmatory and exploratory factor analyses (Erez & Judge, 2001; Judge, Bono, & Locke, 2000; Judge, Locke, Durham, & Kluger, 1998). Moreover, though not considering all four core traits, a few studies have investigated the possibility that the traits may indicate a higher order factor. Specifically, Hunter, Gerbing, and Boster (1982) concluded that self-esteem and locus of control "act like proxies for a second-order factor, which was named self-concept" (p. 1302). Similarly, Hojat (1982) found that self-esteem, locus of control, and neuroticism had their highest loadings on a common factor. Thus, it appears that the four core traits can be treated as measures of the core self-evaluations concept.

TABLE 1
Population Correlations Among Measures of the Four Traits

	Locus of control		Emotional stability		Self-esteem	
	ρ	n	ρ	n	ρ	n
Locus of control	—					
Emotional stability	.40	31	—			
Self-esteem	.52	47	.64	19	—	
Generalized self-efficacy	.56	13	.62	7	.85	9

Note. ρ = population correlation (corrected for measurement error); n = number of studies.

Lack of Discriminant Validity of Core Traits

Discriminant validity refers to differential patterns of correlations of the concepts in question with other variables. In the case of core self-evaluations, this is an issue of whether the four core traits display differential associations with other, theoretically relevant, variables. Because we are using the core traits as measures of the core self-evaluations concept, if the traits showed discriminant validity with other variables, it would weigh *against* the argument that the traits simply are equivalent measures of the same (core self-evaluations) concept. There are at least three theoretically relevant variables that may be used to test if differential relations exist: subjective well-being, job satisfaction, and job performance. DeNeve and Cooper's (1998) meta-analytic results reveal the following with respect to the uncorrected correlation between three of the core traits and subjective well-being: neuroticism, average $r = -.27$; locus of control, average $r = .25$; efficacy, average $r = .23$. With respect to job satisfaction and job performance, Judge and Bono's (2001a) meta-analysis revealed that, with the exception of the correlation between generalized self-efficacy and job satisfaction (which was boosted by a single strong correlation in a one large sample study), the credibility intervals all overlap. Thus, it appears that the core traits do not display much discriminant validity in terms of their correlations with the three outcomes, again supporting the argument that they are indicators of a common concept. Judge, Erez, et al. (2002) further analyzed the discriminant validity of the four traits and found that, in general, the four traits displayed similar patterns of correlations with other variables.

Discriminant Validity Relative to Other Traits

Because core self-evaluations theory posited that emotional stability is an indicator of the broader concept, and emotional stability is one of the most established traits in personality research, it is relevant to ask whether core self-evaluations is simply another label for emotional stability. A separate but related question is how the core self-evaluations concept fits into the five-factor model of personality. As for the first question, at a conceptual level, it appears that emotional stability or neuroticism may be as broad as core self-evaluations. Eysenck's (1990) conceptualization of neuroticism considers self-esteem to be one of the lower order indicators of the concept and Watson and Clark's (1984) conceptualization of negative affectivity, which the authors have subsequently argued is neuroticism (Watson, 2000), also includes self-esteem as one of its indicators. Thus, from a conceptual standpoint, core self-evaluations does not appear to be more broad than emotional stability and, on this basis alone, one might argue that core self-evaluations should be subsumed under the emotional stability concept because the latter has a much more extensive tradition of research.

However, if the core traits and thus core self-evaluations should be subsumed under the label of emotional stability, this does not mean that typical measures of emotional stability adequately represent this broad construct. Typically, measures of neuroticism, perhaps owing to its psychopathological origins, assess dysphoria, hostility, stress, and anxiety. As Judge and Bono (2001b) noted, most measures of neuroticism do not explicitly assess beliefs about one's capabilities or control over one's environment. For example, there are no items in the neuroticism scales of the NEO–FFI (Costa & McCrae, 1992b), the International Personality Item Pool (Goldberg, 1999), or the Eysenck Personality Inventory (Eysenck & Eysenck, 1968) that explicitly reference control or capability. Thus, although core self-evaluations may be no broader than the theoretical concept of neuroticism, we believe that existing measures of neuroticism are too narrow to fully capture self-evaluations.

Another possibility is that the core self-evaluations concept is a broad trait that represents a composite of several Big Five traits (or facets of several traits). To explore the relation of the core traits to the five-factor model, Judge, Erez, et al. (2002) cumulated correlations between the core traits and the Big Five traits. The estimates were corrected for unreliability using reliability estimates reported in Judge, Bono, Ilies, and Gerhardt (2002). The correlations are based on data that Judge and colleagues have collected, as well as several articles that have reported correlations between one of the core traits and the Big Five (Jackson & Gerard, 1996; Kwan, Bond, & Singelis, 1997; Morrison, 1997).

The correlations of the core traits with the Big Five traits are provided in Table 2. As the table shows, each of the core traits correlates the most strongly with neuroticism. Furthermore, these correlations are slightly higher than the average intercorrelation among different measures of the Big Five traits. However, Table 2 also reveals that the core traits correlate moderately strongly with extraversion and conscientiousness. Openness and agreeableness also display nontrivial correlations with the core traits, but in general these correlations are considerably weaker and less consistent than those involving extraversion and conscientiousness. Setting aside neuroticism for the moment, the three core traits

TABLE 2
Relationship of Core Traits to Five-Factor Model of Personality

	Neuroticism	Extraversion	Openness	Agreeableness	Conscientiousness
Neuroticism	—	−.30	−.02	−.29	−.49
Self-esteem	−.66	.42	.23	.20	.46
Locus of control	−.51	.36	.03	.16	.47
Generalized self-efficacy	−.59	.54	.25	.20	.46

Note. Correlations are meta-analytic population correlations (corrected for measurement error).

display an average correlation of .44 with extraversion and .46 with conscientiousness. These are substantial correlations and support the argument that core self-evaluations is a broader concept indicated by (or a composite of) three Big Five traits—neuroticism, conscientiousness, and extraversion.

However, it is important to note that the correlations of the three core traits (self-esteem, locus of control, generalized self-efficacy) with the Big Five traits tend to be similar to the correlations of neuroticism with the other Big Five traits. An examination of Table 2 reveals that the three core traits display stronger correlations with extraversion than neuroticism. However, for conscientiousness and agreeableness, the correlations of the three core traits are actually smaller than the neuroticism–conscientiousness and the neuroticism–agreeableness correlations. On the one hand, core self-evaluations cannot be argued to be independent of extraversion and conscientiousness. On the other hand, although theoretically the Big Five represent five orthogonal personality traits, measures of neuroticism are correlated with measures of conscientiousness and extraversion. Thus, empirically, neither neuroticism nor the other three core traits are independent of extraversion and conscientiousness.

Predictive Validity

Past research has suggested that the individual core traits are related to both performance and job satisfaction. In terms of job performance, Judge and Bono's (2001b) meta-analytic results suggest that the individual core traits show validities that are quite comparable to the validity of individual measure of conscientiousness. Specifically, the average validity of the four core traits in predicting job performance was .23 in Judge and Bono's (2001a) meta-analysis, which is identical to the average validity Barrick and Mount (1991) found for conscientiousness. When traits are considered at the construct level (e.g., when conscientiousness or the four core traits are aggregated to an overall construct), again, the validity levels are roughly comparable—.30 for core self-evaluations (Judge, Erez, et al. 2002) and .31 for conscientiousness (Mount & Barrick, 1995). Much has been made of the validity of conscientiousness as a predictor of job performance. These results suggest that another trait, core self-evaluations, should be placed alongside conscientiousness as a valid personality predictor of job performance. Equally important, the results suggest that when the traits are viewed as an indicator of a common concept, validity increases rather dramatically.

If the core self-evaluations concept is an important predictor of job performance, how is it so? Judge, Erez, and Bono (1998) argued that the core self-evaluations concept should influence performance mainly through its effect on motivation. According to these authors, several theories of motivation might explain the effect of core self-evaluations on performance. Erez and Judge (2001) conducted two studies to investigate the degree to which motivation mediated the relation between core self-evaluations and performance. In a laboratory study, Erez and Judge found that the core self-evaluations factor was positively related to self-reported task motivation ($r = .39, p < .01$), an objective measure of task persistence ($r = .24, p < .05$), and task performance ($r = .35, p < .01$). In a second study, a field study of insurance agents, Erez and Judge found that the core self-evaluations factor was positively related to sales goal level ($r = .42, p < .01$), goal commitment ($r = .59, p < .01$), and both objective (sales volume; $r = .35, p < .01$) and supervisory ratings ($r = .44, p < .01$) of job performance. In both studies, Erez and Judge found that motivation mediated about half of the relation between core self-evaluations and performance. Thus, it appears that core self-evaluations is a motivational trait and this explains much of its effect on job performance.

In addition to job performance, core self-evaluations is related to job satisfaction. Judge and Bono's (2001a) meta-analysis of the relation of the four individual core traits to job satisfaction revealed an average correlation of .32 between the four individual core traits and job satisfaction. When these traits were aggregated, however, this correlation increases substantially to .41. Judge and Heller (2002) found that core self-evaluations was more strongly related to job satisfaction than was positive and negative affectivity or the Big Five traits. Thus, the core self-evaluations concept is perhaps the best dispositional predictor of job satisfaction.

Why is the core self-evaluations concept consistently related to job satisfaction? Two studies have suggested one explanation—intrinsic job characteristics mediate the relation between core self-evaluations and job satisfaction. By intrinsic job characteristics, we mean the Hackman and Oldham (1980) core job dimensions (task identity, skill variety, task significance, autonomy, and feedback). In three studies and across various specifications, Judge, Locke, et al. (1998) showed that roughly 37% of the influence of core self-evaluations on job satisfaction was mediated by perceptions of intrinsic job characteristics. Although the Judge, Locke, et al. study helped to illuminate the process by which core self-evaluations influenced job satisfaction, the studies used only perceptual measures of job characteristics. It is not clear from Judge, Locke, et al.'s findings to what degree the core self-evaluations concept is related to increased job complexity as opposed (or in addition) to enhanced perceptions of work characteristics. Accordingly, Judge et al. (2000) tested the mediating role of job characteristics using both objective (coding job titles using the Dictionary Occupational Titles job complexity scoring) and perceptual measures of job characteristics. In two studies, their results indicated that core self-evaluations was related to the actual attainment of complex jobs as well as to the perceptual measures of job characteristics (holding objective complexity constant). Thus, it appears that core self-evaluations influences job satisfaction, in part, because positive individuals actually obtain more challenging jobs, and also because they perceive jobs of equal complexity as more intrinsically fulfilling.

If the arguments presented earlier in the article regarding correspondence are correct and applicable to core self-evaluations, then the broad core trait should predict broad criteria better than the individual traits. We should note that the bandwidth-fidelity issue is currently being debated in both the personality and the personnel selection literatures, with advocates on all sides of the issue (see Costa & McCrae, 1992a; Eysenck, 1992; John, Hampson, & Goldberg, 1991; Ones & Viswesvaran, 1996; Schneider, Hough, & Dunnette, 1996). Our specific concern here is the relative predictive validity of the broad core self-evaluations concept versus the four specific traits. Erez and Judge (2001) have addressed this issue explicitly in terms of the relation of core self-evaluations to motivation and job performance. They found that the overall core concept always predicted motivation and performance, whereas the individual traits did so inconsistently. Judge, Erez, et al. (2002) also demonstrated that the core factor better predicted criteria (job satisfaction, life satisfaction) than did the individual core traits. Thus, it appears that the overall concept is a more consistent predictor of outcomes than are the individual traits.

MEASUREMENT OF CORE SELF-EVALUATIONS

Despite support for the concept of core self-evaluations, one limiting issue is the measurement of the trait. Most traits are measured directly. For example, the best-known measures of conscientiousness measure the trait with scales that consist of 9 to 12 items (Benet-Martínez & John, 1998; Costa & McCrae, 1992b; Goldberg, 1999). In contrast, core self-evaluations have been measured indirectly, with relatively lengthy scales (e.g., Judge et al., 2000; Judge, Locke, et al., 1998). This measurement strategy has several limitations.

First, the measures are indirect. This means that the core self-evaluations trait must be extracted by factor analyzing the four scales that indicate the trait (e.g., Judge, Erez, et al., 1998). A direct measure, because it is designed to precisely measure the underlying concept itself, rather than the indicators of the concept, may be more valid. The indirect measurement approach of past research also leads to confusion over whether the trait is a latent or aggregate construct (see later). Second, because of this indirect measurement from existing scales, the measure of core self-evaluations is relatively long. Judge, Locke, et al. (1998) and Judge et al. (2000) measured core self-evaluations with four scales that total 38 items. Given the relative brevity of measures of other traits, it would seem unnecessary to measure core self-evaluations with a combination of scales that, cumulatively, are relatively long. The length of the indirect measure may limit its usefulness, especially in organizational settings. Rather than utilizing a lengthy measure, some researchers may choose to measure only a single indicator (e.g., neuroticism or emotional stability) and thereby miss a substantial amount of valid variance. A final possible limitation is that of empirical validity. The core traits display slightly differential relations with criterion variables (e.g., in Judge & Bono's, 2001a, meta-analysis, emotional stability predicted the criteria less well than the other core traits, and the self-esteem-performance correlations were highly variable across studies); it is possible that a direct measure would achieve higher, and less variable, levels of validity.

Accordingly, Judge, Erez, Bono, and Thoresen (2003) developed and validated a direct measure of core self-evaluations, which they termed the Core Self-Evaluations Scale (CSES). This measure consists of 12 items and is provided in Table 3. To test the validity of the measure, four independent samples were collected. Their results suggested that the measure is reliable, as assessed by internal consistency (average $\alpha = .84$) and test–retest reliability ($r = .81$ over a 3-month period). Furthermore, the inter-source (self–significant other) level of agreement was comparable to that of other personality measures. For example, the self and peer reports for the CSES were correlated $r = .43$, a level of convergence similar to that typically obtained in research with established Big Five measures (Barbaranelli & Caprara, 2000; Costa & McCrae, 1992b; Mount, Barrick, & Strauss, 1994). Factor-analytic results also suggested that the 12 CSES items loaded on a single dimensional construct.

Furthermore, the CSES displayed convergent validity as evidenced by its correlations with the four core traits. Second, it was significantly correlated with job satisfaction, life satisfaction, and supervisory ratings of job performance and dis-

TABLE 3
The Core Self-Evaluations Scale (CSES)

Instructions: Following are several statements about you with which you may agree or disagree. Using the response scale provided, indicate your agreement or disagreement with each item by placing the appropriate number on the line preceding that item.

> 1 = Strongly disagree
> 2 = Disagree
> 3 = Neutral
> 4 = Agree
> 5 = Strongly agree

_____ I am confident I get the success I deserve in life.
_____ Sometimes I feel depressed. (reverse-scored)
_____ When I try, I generally succeed.
_____ Sometimes when I fail I feel worthless. (reverse-scored)
_____ I complete tasks successfully.
_____ Sometimes, I do not feel in control of my work. (reverse-scored)
_____ Overall, I am satisfied with myself.
_____ I am filled with doubts about my competence. (reverse-scored)
_____ I determine what will happen in my life.
_____ I do not feel in control of my success in my career. (reverse-scored)
_____ I am capable of coping with most of my problems.
_____ There are times when things look pretty bleak and hopeless to me. (reverse- scored)

played incremental validity in predicting these criteria controlling for the core self-evaluations factor as well as the traits from the five-factor model. Judge et al. (in press) noted that the CSES may be labeled a measure of emotional stability. If so, the CSES should prove useful in future research on emotional stability.

Cross-Cultural Evidence of the Core Self-Evaluations Scale

Personality constructs, such as the Five-Factor Model, have been extensively examined across different countries and languages, to find further evidence for their cross-cultural robustness (Benet-Martinez & John, 1998; McCrae & Costa, 1997). To date, no such cross-cultural comparison has been made with the CSES. In this article, we report some findings concerning the psychometric properties and validities of Spanish and Dutch versions of the CSES as studied with samples from Spain and The Netherlands. The validities of the scales were examined through correlating them with the Big Five dimensions (discriminant validity) and through relating them to job relevant variables; that is, job satisfaction and career ambition (predictive validity).

The data were collected from three independent samples, one student sample from Spain (Sample 1), one student sample from The Netherlands (Sample 2), and employees of an insurance company (Sample 3) from The Netherlands. In all three samples, we collected data on the CSES items. Moreover, in one of the student samples (Sample 1), we collected data on career ambition; in the field sample (Sample 3), we collected data on the Big Five personality traits and job satisfaction. The three samples allow us to examine the psychometric properties of the CSES. Both the field sample and the Spanish student samples allow us to investigate various aspects of the validity of the CSES.

Participants in Sample 1 were undergraduates enrolled at a Spanish university. Participants completed a questionnaire in a classroom session as a pretest for a lab experiment. A total of 427 individuals completed the CSES questionnaire and the questions concerning their career ambition. Participant ages ranged from 18 to 34 years ($M = 20.9$, $SD = 2.2$); 55% were women. Participants in Sample 2 were undergraduates at a Dutch university. They received course credit for their participation. There were 509 participants with an average age of 21.5 years ($SD = 5.4$); 70% of participants were women. Participants completed the self-report surveys in a classroom setting. Sample 3 consisted of employees from a large insurance company in The Netherlands. A total of 190 employees from the organization were surveyed about their organizational climate and aspects of their job. In total, 99 employees returned usable survey packets, for a response rate of 52%. The mean age of respondents was 37.2 years ($SD = 9.4$) and respondents reported being employed in their current positions for an average of 6.4 years ($SD = 9.0$). Fifty seven percent of the respondents were men.

Core self-evaluations.   Core self-evaluations were measured with the Core Self-Evaluations Scale (Judge et al., in press). The 12 items of the CSES were translated into Spanish and Dutch. The psychometric properties of the Spanish and Dutch CSES are presented in the results section.

The Big Five traits.   The Big Five traits were measured in Sample 3. We used 60 items derived from the Five-Factor Personality Inventory (FFPI; Hendriks, Hofstee, & De Raad, 1999). The FFPI results from the Abridged Big-Five Dimensional Circumplex taxonomic model of traits (Hofstee, De Raad, & Goldberg, 1992). The five scales (Neuroticism, Extraversion, Openness, Agreeableness and Conscientiousness) showed good reliabilities, ranging from .89 to .93 in previous studies with $N = 1311$. The FFPI also showed good convergent validities with the 225-item trait-adjective rating list and the Revised NEO Personality Inventory (Hendriks, 1997, p. 70). In this study, the coefficient alpha (α) reliabilities of the scales were .80 (Neuroticism), .85 (Extraversion), .84 (Autonomy), .72 (Agreeableness), and .77 (Conscientiousness).

Career ambition.   Career ambition was measured in Sample 1. Three items were derived from the Ambition for a Managerial Position Scale (Van Vianen, 1999), reflecting individuals' intention to fulfill a top position in the future, to have a high-status position, and to strive for making promotions in their job. The reliability of the scale was .77.

Job satisfaction.   Job satisfaction was measured in Sample 3 using five items from the Brayfield and Rothe (1951) measure of overall job satisfaction. The reliability for this scale was .82.

Psychometric properties of the Spanish and Dutch CSES.   Table 4 presents descriptive statistics on the CSES, as well as reliability estimates, across the data sets. As shown in Table 4, the distribution of the CSES was similar across the samples. The means ranged from 3.61 to 3.71 with an average of 3.68 and the standard deviations ranged from .51 to .58 with an average of .54. None of the means were significantly different from one another. Across the three measurements, all coefficient alpha reliability estimates were greater than .80 with an average reliability of .83. These results are similar to the ones that were found with the English version of the CSES (Judge et al., in press). Confirmatory factor analysis, conducted using LISREL 8.50 (Jöreskog & Sörbom, 2001), was used to test the underlying structure of the Spanish and Dutch scales. A variance–covariance matrix was entered as input into the program. The individual items of the scale served as indicators of one latent variable. Three separate tests of the factor structure of the CSES (for each sample) were conducted. To test the fit of the one-factor model, we report the following fit statistics: chi-square (χ^2) with corresponding degrees of

TABLE 4

Descriptive Statistics and Zero-Order Correlations Between the Core Self-Evaluation Scale (CSES), the Five-Factor Model of Personality, Job Satisfaction, and Career Ambition

Sample	M	SD	Internal Consistency	Neuroticism	Extraversion	Openness	Agreeableness	Conscientiousness	Job Satisfaction	Career Ambition
1	3.61	.54	.82	—	—	—	—	—		.29**
2	3.71	.58	.84	—	—	—	—	—	.56**	—
3	3.73	.51	.82	-.66**	.36**	.32**	.23*	.34**	—	—

Note. $^{*}p < .05$ (two tailed test); $^{**}p < .01$ (two tailed test).

freedom, Root-Mean-Square Residual, Root-Mean-Square Error of Approximation, Goodness-of-Fit Index, Comparative Fit Index, Relative Fit Index, and the average factor loading of the items on the factor. The fit statistics for the single factor
model are reported in Table 5. These fit statistics represented a good fit of the hypothesized model to the data across the three samples and suggest that the CSES
items are indicators of a single latent construct. Moreover, the fit indexes are in ac-
cordance with those that were found with the English version of the CSES (Judge
et al., in press).

Indicators of validity.   Table 4 presents the correlations of the CSES with the
Big Five dimensions as measured with Sample 3. As in the Judge et al. (in press)
study, we expected the CSES to be correlated with conscientiousness and
extraversion (see also Judge & Bono, 2001b). As shown in Table 4, both conscientiousness ($r = .34, p < .01$) and extraversion ($r = .36, p < .01$) were moderately correlated with CSES. Judge et al. (in press) found weak links between the core traits
and the other Big Five traits, agreeableness and openness. However, as Table 4
shows, the relations of the CSES with Agreeableness and Openness in our sample
were more substantial (agreeableness: $r = .23, p < .05$; openness: $r = .32, p < .01$).
The moderate correlation with openness is likely to be the result of the different
content of this scale (i.e., it rather refers to autonomy) as compared to the openness
scale of the NEO-PI-R. As expected, we found a high negative correlation between
the CSES and neuroticism ($r = -.66, p < .01$). These results suggest that the Dutch
CSES is a valid construct inasmuch as it strongly converges with neuroticism and
moderately converges with conscientiousness and extraversion, according to previous findings with the English CSES. We tested the predictive validity of the
Dutch CSES using job satisfaction as the criterion and we tested the predictive va-

TABLE 5
Fit Statistics from Confirmatory Factor Analysis of Single Dimensional
Structure of the Spanish and Dutch Core Self-Evaluations Scales (CSES)

Fit Statistic	Spanish CSES Students	Dutch CSES Students	Employees
Chi-square (χ^2)	88.92	168.83	75.24
Degrees of freedom	50	50	50
Root mean square residual	.03	.05	.06
Root mean square error of approximation	.04	.07	.08
Goodness of fit index	.97	.95	.88
Comparative fit index	.96	.93	.91
Relative fit index	.90	.88	.72
Average factor loading	.52	.54	.52

Note.   [a]$N = 427$. [b]$N = 509$. [c]$N = 99$.

lidity of the Spanish CSES using career ambition as the criterion. Past research found the core self-evaluation construct to be related to job satisfaction (Erez & Judge, 2001; Judge & Bono, 2001a; Judge et al., 2000; Judge, Locke, et al., 1998). Table 4 shows that in Sample 3 the Dutch CSES was strongly and positively correlated with job satisfaction ($r = .56, p < .01$). We already argued that core self-evaluations are a motivational trait. Career ambition can be conceived of as the motivation to move forward in one's career. Moreover, Judge et al. (2000) showed that individuals with positive self-evaluations obtained more challenging jobs. Therefore, we examined the relation between career ambition and the Spanish CSES. Table 4 shows a significant moderate correlation between career ambition and the Spanish CSES ($r = .29, p < .01$).

To summarize, the results with the Spanish and Dutch versions of the CSES corroborate those that were found with the original English version of the CSES concerning their psychometric properties and some indicators of validity. Future cross-cultural studies should further establish their test–retest reliabilities and should provide more evidence for their predictive validities.

AN AGENDA FOR FUTURE RESEARCH

Because of the development of the core self-evaluation concept (Judge et al., 1997), considerable research has been performed that supported the existence of core self-evaluations as a higher order factor of self-esteem, emotional stability, generalized self-efficacy, and locus of control. Moreover, several indicators of its validity have been thoroughly tested and core self-evaluations proved to be a better predictor than each of its underlying traits. Finally, a direct measure of CSES has been developed and has been found to be reliable and valid.

The core self-evaluations construct is a promising one and might induce abundant research in diverse research areas. However, some issues concerning the core self-evaluations are not yet addressed and need to be the focus of future research. Later, we discuss some of these research themes.

Two Indicators of Emotional Stability

If the argument is that there are two main indicators of emotional stability—one that may be termed anxiety and another that may be termed depressive self-concept (or positive core evaluations in the positive)—this hypothesis needs to be documented in future research. The first step would be to determine whether such a structure can be confirmed via confirmatory factor analysis. The second step would be to show that these two indicators display differential patterns of correlations with theoretically relevant variables. Specifically, the anxiety aspect of emotional stability would be expected to correlate more highly with stress and strain and the depressive aspect would be expected to correlate more highly with criteria such as job satisfaction, life satisfaction, and job performance.

Person-Centered and Circumplex Approaches to Personality

The validity of personality dimensions has traditionally been examined through predicting job criteria from single personality constructs. This variable-centered approach toward predictive validity focuses on personality differences between individuals rather than on the clustering of personality variables within individuals (i.e., a person-centered approach). Although core self-evaluations comprises a clustering of four traits, the construct has been developed from a variable-centered perspective. The four traits are perceived as belonging to a single higher order concept rather than reflecting a personality pattern within individuals. A person-centered approach was recently used in a study of De Fruyt (2002), in which he identified two groups of individuals with similar personality patterns through cluster analyzing individuals' NEO–PI–R scores. The first group included individuals with relatively high scores on neuroticism and relatively low scores on extraversion and conscientiousness. The second group comprised individuals with relatively low scores on neuroticism and relatively high scores on conscientiousness. Individuals of the first group were significantly more unemployed and—if employed—less satisfied with their job and experienced more stress than individuals of the second group. Additionally, circumplex approaches to trait structures (see Hofstee et al., 1992) suggest the existence of specific facets combining levels of neuroticism with levels of each of the other Big Five traits. When applying these circumplex models to core self-evaluations and Big Five traits, a more fine-tuned framework of job-related personality typologies might emerge. Furthermore, future studies should examine if these personality typologies (i.e., the constellation of core self-evaluations and Big Five traits) could further increase the predictive validity of personality measures.

Stability of Core Self-Evaluations

In work and organizational psychology, there is a longstanding dispositional–situational controversy. The dispositional approach proposes that individuals possess stable traits that significantly influence their affective and behavioral reactions to organizational settings (Davis-Blake & Pfeffer, 1989). Individual differences in personality traits are considered to be extremely stable in adults, even over periods of as long as three decades, during which most people will have experienced major life changes (McCrae, 2002). Others questioned the importance of dispositions and took a situational perspective for explaining (differences in) organizational behavior. The situational approach proposes that individuals are highly responsive and adaptive to organizational settings and that personality traits change in response to organizational settings (Davis-Blake & Pfeffer, 1989). McCrae (2002), however, noted that personality changes associated with environmental influences are difficult to assess because of ambiguity of the causal direction, small sample-sizes and the lack of replication of the findings.

So far, only one study examined the stability (over a 3-month period) of core self-evaluations (Judge et al., in press). More research has been done concerning the stability of its underlying constructs (i.e., neuroticism and self-esteem). Neuroticism is considered a relatively stable personality construct (e.g., Costa & McCrae, 1988; McCrae, 1993). To illustrate, Costa and McCrae (1988) found a 6-year stability coefficient of .82. Furthermore, a study done on moderator variables of stability in personality (including neuroticism) led them to conclude that "These findings confirm the view that personality traits are extremely stable in adulthood and that uncorrected stability coefficients, even those as high as .80, underestimate true stability" (McCrae, 1993, p. 583).

Self-esteem is generally assumed to be a stable trait. However, Trzesniewski, Donnellan, and Robins (2003) recently showed that the stability of self-esteem is relatively low during early childhood, increases throughout adolescence and young adulthood, and than declines during midlife and old-age. They concluded that, because substantial levels of continuity across decades of life were found, self-esteem is best to be characterized as showing both continuity and change across the life span (p. 216). Moreover, some researchers not only consider the implications of the level of self-esteem, but also the (in)stability of self-esteem of importance. Kernis, Cornell, Sun, Berry, and Harlow (1993), for instance, stated:

> It has also become clear that people differ in the extent to which they exhibit short-term fluctuations in their contextually based self-esteem (i.e., stability of self-esteem). Most important, recent research indicates that differences between and within high and low self-esteem individuals (SEs) emerge as a function of stability of self-esteem. (p. 1190)

Research on the stability of core self-evaluations will have to answer the question with regard to the stability of this construct.

Although the stability of traits is an important issue, the question whether dispositions can be changed is not fully answered by showing their stability. Environmental influences that are intense, sustained, and/or deliberately designed may induce small but meaningful personality changes over time (McCrae, 2002). Because the core self-evaluations are related to highly appreciated work outcomes like motivation, job satisfaction, and job performance, the malleability of the core self-evaluation is an issue worthy of future attention.

Self versus Other Ratings

Past research has utilized self versus other ratings of core self-evaluations (Judge et al., in press). This raises the interesting question of whether individuals can be too positive in their self-assessment. In the leadership literature, London (2002) has discussed the role of self-insight and whether self-other discrepancies in leadership ratings reflect overestimates or underestimates of the leader. Though defining reality in such a context may not be a productive pursuit, it does raise the question of whether one can be too positive in one's self-assessment. Baumeister, Campbell, Krueger, and Vohs (2003) commented in a recent review, "Perhaps it is more valuable and adaptive to understand oneself honestly and accurately, even when this means feeling bad about oneself" (p. 38). In the context of core self-evaluations, can one be too positive for one's own (or other's) good? This would be an interesting and important area for future research.

States and Traits

Related to the aforementioned, it is not unusual for the individual core traits to be treated as dependent variables in the various literatures in which they are studied. This is particularly true for the core trait that seems to be at the center of core self-evaluations: self-esteem. For example, Keltikangas-Jaervinen, Kivimaeki, and Keskivaara (2003) investigated the effect of parental child-rearing practices on self-esteem; MacMaster, Donovan, and MacIntyre (2002) studied the effect of childhood disability on self-esteem; and Bizman and Yinon (2002) investigated the effect of the outcomes of athletic contests on self-esteem. There is evidence to suggest that the heritability of the individual core traits is comparable to that of measures of neuroticism (Judge & Bono, 2001a). However, self-esteem has often been used as a dependent variable and, hence, one may wonder whether, and to what degree, core self-evaluations is malleable and influenced by the situation.

CONCLUSION

In this article we have presented a review of core self-evaluations research. Although introduction of the term is relatively new, because it is a latent concept that is indicated by some of the more commonly investigated traits in psychology, its origins are not new. We have presented a review of core self-evaluations research, introduced some new research on the first direct measure of the concept, and suggested some new areas for future research. We believe the concept is, along with conscientiousness, the most useful personality trait in the realm of human performance.

REFERENCES

Barbaranelli, C., & Caprara, G. V. (2000). Measuring the Big Five in self-report and other ratings: A multitrait–multimethod study. *European Journal of Psychological Assessment, 16,* 31–43.

Barrick, M. R., & Mount, M. K. (1991). The Big Five personality dimensions and job performance: A meta-analysis. *Personnel Psychology, 44,* 1–26.

Barrick, M. R., Mount, M. K., & Judge, T. A. (2001). Personality and performance at the beginning of the new millennium: What do we know and where do we go next? *International Journal of Selection & Assessment, 9,* 9–30.

Baumeister, R. F., Campbell, J. D., Krueger, J. I., & Vohs, K. D. (2003). Does high self-esteem cause better performance, interpersonal success, happiness, or healthier lifestyles? *Psychological Science in the Public Interest, 4,* 1–44.

Benet-Martínez, V., & John, O. P. (1998). *Los Cinco Grandes* across cultures and ethnic groups: Multitrait-multimethod analyses of the Big Five in Spanish and English. *Journal of Personality and Social Psychology, 75,* 729–750.

Bizman, A., & Yinon, Y. (2002). Engaging in distancing tactics among sport fans: Effects on self-esteem and emotional responses. *Journal of Social Psychology, 142,* 381–392.

Brayfield, A. H., & Rothe, H. F. (1951). An index of job satisfaction. *Journal of Applied Psychology, 35,* 307–311.

Brockner, J. (1979). The effects of self-esteem. Success-failure, and self-consciousness on task performance. *Journal of Personality and Social Psychology, 37,* 1732–1741.

Costa, P. T., & McCrae, R. R (1988). Personality in adulthood: A six-year longitudinal study of self-reports and spouse ratings on the NEO Personality Inventory. *Journal of Personality and Social Psychology, 54,* 853–863.

Costa, P. T., & McCrae, R. R. (1992a). Four ways five factors are basic. *Personality and Individual Differences, 13,* 653–665.

Costa, P. T., Jr., & McCrae, R. (1992b). *NEO–PI–R and NEO–FFI professional manual.* Odessa, FL: Psychological Assessment Resources.

Davis-Blake, A., & Pfeffer, J. (1989). Just a mirage: The search for dispositional effects in organizational research. *Academy of Management Review, 14,* 385–400.

De Fruyt, F. (2002). A person-centered approach to P–E fit questions using a multiple trait model. *Journal of Vocational Behavior, 60,* 73–90.

DeNeve, K. M., & Cooper, H. (1998). The happy personality: A meta-analysis of 137 personality traits and subjective well-being. *Psychological Bulletin, 124,* 197–229.

Dewey, R. (1974). Six pillars of the social sciences' Tower of Babel. *Etc.: A Review of General Semantics, 31,* 239–247.

Erez, A., & Judge, T. A. (2001). Relationship of core self-evaluations to goal setting, motivation, and performance. *Journal of Applied Psychology, 86,* 1270–1279.

Eysenck, H. J. (1990). Biological dimensions of personality. In L. A. Pervin (Ed.), *Handbook of personality* (pp. 244–276). New York: Guilford.

Eysenck, H. J. (1992). Four ways five factors are *not* basic. *Personality and Individual Differences, 13,* 667–673.

Eysenck, H. J., & Eysenck, S. B. G. (1968). *Manual for the Eysenck Personality Inventory.* San Diego, CA: Educational and Industrial Testing Service.

Francis, L. J. (1996). The relationship between Rosenberg's construct of self-esteem and Eysenck's two-dimensional model of personality. *Personality and Individual Differences, 21,* 483–488.

Freud, S. (1910). The origin and development of psychoanalysis. *American Journal of Psychology, 21,* 181–218.

Furnham, A., & Zacherl, M. (1986). Personality and job satisfaction. *Personality and Individual Differences, 7,* 453–459.

Goldberg, L. R. (1999). A broad-bandwidth, public-domain, personality inventory measuring the lower-level facets of several five-factor models. In I. Mervielde, I. J. Deary, F. De Fruyt, & F. Ostendorf (Eds.), *Personality psychology in Europe* (Vol. 7, pp. 7–28). Tilburg, The Netherlands: Tilburg University Press.

Hackman, J., & Oldham, G. (1980). *Work redesign.* Reading, MA: Addison-Wesley.

Hendriks, A. A. (1997). *The construction of the Five-Factor Personality Inventory (FFPI).* Unpublished doctoral dissertation, University of Groningen, The Netherlands.

Hendriks, A. A. J., Hofstee, W. K. B., & De Raad, B. (1999). The Five-Factor Personality Inventory (FFPI). *Personality and Individual Differences, 27,* 307–325.

Hjelle, L. A., & Clouser, R. (1970). Susceptibility to attitude change as a function of internal–external control. *Psychological Record, 20,* 305–310.

Hofstee, W. K. B., De Raad, B., & Goldberg, L. R. (1992). Integration of the Big Five and circumplex approaches to trait structure. *Journal of Personality and Social Psychology, 63,* 146–163.

Hojat, M. (1982). Loneliness as a function of selected personality variables. *Journal of Clinical Psychology, 38,* 137–141.

Hunter, J. E., Gerbing, D. W., & Boster, F. J. (1982). Machiavellian beliefs and personality: Construct validity of the Machiavellianism dimension. *Journal of Personality and Social Psychology, 43,* 1293–1305.

Jackson, L. A., & Gerard, D. A. (1996). Diurnal types, the "Big Five" personality factors, and other personal characteristics. *Journal of Social Behavior and Personality, 11,* 273–283.

John, O. P., Hampson, S. E., & Goldberg, L. R. (1991). The basic level in personality–trait hierarchies: Studies of trait use and accessibility in different contexts. *Journal of Personality and Social Psychology, 60,* 348–361.

Jöreskog, K., & Sörbom, D. (2001). *LISREL 8.50: User's reference guide.* Chicago: Scientific Software International.

Judge, T. A., & Bono, J. E. (2001a). Relationship of core self-evaluations traits—self-esteem, generalized self-efficacy, locus of control, and emotional stability—with job satisfaction and job performance: A meta-analysis. *Journal of Applied Psychology, 86,* 80–92.

Judge, T. A., & Bono, J. E. (2001b). A rose by any other name... Are self-esteem, generalized self-efficacy, neuroticism, and locus of control indicators of a common construct? In B. W. Roberts, & R. Hogan (Eds.), *Personality psychology in the workplace* (pp. 93–118). Washington, DC: American Psychological Association.

Judge, T. A., Bono, J. E., Erez, A., Locke, E. A., & Thoresen, C. J. (2002). The scientific merit of valid measures of general concepts: Personality research and core self-evaluation. In J. Brett & F. Dragow (Eds.), The psychology of work: Theoretically based empirical research (pp. 55–77). Mahwah, NJ: Lawrence Erlbaum Associates, Inc.

Judge, T. A., Bono, J. E., Ilies, R., & Gerhardt, M. (2002). Personality and leadership: A qualitative and quantitative review. *Journal of Applied Psychology, 87,* 765–780.

Judge, T. A., Bono, J. E., & Locke, E. A. (2000). Personality and job satisfaction: The mediating role of job characteristics. *Journal of Applied Psychology, 85,* 237–249.

Judge, T. A., Erez, A., & Bono, J. E. (1998). The power of being positive: The relationship between positive self-concept and job performance. *Human Performance, 11,* 167–187.

Judge, T. A., Erez, A., Bono, J. E., & Thoresen, C. J. (2002). Are measures of self-esteem, neuroticism, locus of control, and generalized self-efficacy indicators of a common core construct? *Journal of Personality and Social Psychology, 83,* 693–710.

Judge, T. A., Erez, A., Bono, J. E., & Thoresen, C. J. (2003). The Core Self-Evaluations Scale (CSES): Development of a measure. *Personnel Psychology.*

Judge, T. A., & Heller, D. (2002, April). The dispositional sources of job satisfaction: An integrative test. In R. Ilies & T. A. Judge (Chairs), *Dispositional influences on work-related attitudes.* Symposium presentation at the Society for Industrial and Organizational Psychology Annual Meetings, Toronto.

Judge, T. A., Locke, E. A., & Durham, C. C. (1997). The dispositional causes of job satisfaction: A core evaluations approach. *Research in Organizational Behavior, 19,* 151–188.

Judge, T. A., Locke, E. A., Durham, C. C., & Kluger, A. N. (1998). Dispositional effects on job and life satisfaction: The role of core evaluations. *Journal of Applied Psychology, 83,* 17–34.

Keltikangas-Jaervinen, L., Kivimaeki, M., & Keskivaara, P. (2003). Parental practices, self-esteem and adult temperament: 17-year follow-up study of four population-based age cohorts. *Personality and Individual Differences, 34,* 431–447.

Kernis, M. H., Cornell, D. P., Sun, C. R., Berry, A., & Harlow, T. (1993). There's more to self-esteem than whether it is high or low: The importance of stability of self-esteem. *Journal of Personality and Social Psychology, 65,* 1190–1204.

Kwan, V. S. Y., Bond, M. H., & Singelis, T. M. (1997). Pancultural explanations for life satisfaction: Adding relationship harmony to self-esteem. *Journal of Personality and Social Psychology, 73,* 1038–1051.

London, M. (2002). *Leadership development: Paths to self-insight and professional growth.* Mahwah, NJ: Lawrence Erlbaum Associates, Inc.

MacMaster, K., Donovan, L. A., & MacIntyre, P. D. (2002). The effects of being diagnosed with a learning disability on children's self-esteem. *Child Study Journal, 32,* 101–108.

McCrae, R. R. (1993). Moderated analyses of longitudinal personality stability. *Journal of Personality and Social Psychology, 65,* 577–585.

McCrae, R. R. (2002). The maturation of personality psychology: Adult personality development and psychological well-being. *Journal of Research in Personality, 36,* 307–317.

McCrae, R. R., & Costa, P. T. (1997). Personality trait structure as a human universal. *American Psychologist, 52,* 509–516.

Morrison, K. A. (1997). Personality correlates of the five-factor model for a sample of business owners/managers: Associations with scores on self-monitoring, Type A behavior, locus of control, and subjective well-being. *Psychological Reports, 80,* 255–272.

Mount, M. K., & Barrick, M. R. (1995). The Big Five personality dimensions: Implications for research and practice in human resources management. *Research in Personnel and Human Resources Management, 13,* 153–200.

Mount, M. K., Barrick, M. R., & Strauss, J. P. (1994). Validity of observer ratings of the Big Five personality factors. *Journal of Applied Psychology, 79,* 272–280.

Ones, D. S. (1993). *The construct validity of integrity tests.* Unpublished doctoral dissertation, University of Iowa.

Ones, D. S., Mount, M. K., Barrick, M. R., & Hunter, J. E. (1994). Personality and job performance: A critique of the Tett, Jackson, and Rothstein (1991) meta-analysis. *Personnel Psychology, 47,* 147–156.

Ones, D. S., & Viswesvaran, C. (1996). Bandwidth-fidelity dilemma in personality measurement for personnel selection. *Journal of Organizational Behavior, 17,* 609–626.

Salgado, J. F. (1997). The five factor model of personality and job performance in the European Community. *Journal of Applied Psychology, 82,* 30–43.

Schneider, R. J., Hough, L. M., & Dunnette, M. D. (1996). Broadsided by broad traits: How to sink science in five dimensions or less. *Journal of Organizational Behavior, 17,* 639–655.

Schwab, D. P. (1980). Construct validity in organizational behavior. *Research in Organizational Behavior, 2,* 3–43.

Smith, C. A., Organ, D. W., & Near, J. P. (1983). Organizational citizenship behavior: Its nature and antecedents. *Journal of Applied Psychology, 68,* 653–663.

Tett, R. P., Jackson, D. N., & Rothstein, M. (1991). Personality measures as predictors of job performance: A meta-analytic review. *Personnel Psychology, 44,* 703–742.

Tokar, D. M., & Subich, L. M. (1997). Relative contributions of congruence and personality dimensions to job satisfaction. *Journal of Vocational Behavior, 50,* 482–491.

Trzesniewski, K. H., Donnellan, M. B., & Robins, R. W. (2003). Stability of self-esteem across the life span. *Journal of Personality & Social Psychology, 84,* 205–220.

Van Vianen, A. E. M. (1999). Managerial self-efficacy, outcome expectations, and work-role salience as determinants of ambition for a managerial position. *Journal of Applied Social Psychology, 29,* 639–655.

Watson, D. (2000). *Mood and temperament.* New York: Guilford.

Watson, D., & Clark, L. A. (1984). Negative affectivity: The disposition to experience aversive emotional states. *Psychological Bulletin, 96,* 465–490.

HUMAN PERFORMANCE, *17*(3), 347–357

Beyond the Big Five: Increases in Understanding and Practical Utility

Neal Schmitt

Department of Psychology
Michigan State University

The articles in this special issue provide presentations of measures of three new personality constructs. Initial results from these three programs of research indicate that each of these measures has a firm theoretical base and that the authors have engaged in careful consideration of the set of relations that theory suggests ought to be displayed by their new measure. Further empirical research by these authors and others ought to provide greater scientific understanding of the role personality plays in work satisfaction and various dimensions of performance, a better sense of the practical usefulness of these measures, and better information about the situational constraints that apply when each is used to predict various personal and organizational outcomes.

It is almost obligatory in articles on personality to cite the work of two previous research teams. One is the work of Guion and Gottier (1965), in which the authors supposedly ended personality research for three decades because of their gloomy view of the validity of personality measures. The second is the work of Costa and McRae (1988), who presented the view that the myriad of personality measures available really represent five underlying constructs. The three articles in this special issue of *Human Performance* challenge those early conclusions and extend that work. They represent a welcome departure from the type of research on the validity of the Big Five that seems to have become commonplace in the last 15 years.

Meta-analytic work (Barrick & Mount, 1991) challenged the Guion and Gottier conclusion that validity research on the use of personality measures did not warrant their use in predicting job performance. Guion and Gottier were right on one point, however; observed validities of personality measures then

---

Requests for reprints should be sent to Neal Schmitt, Department of Psychology, Michigan State University, East Lansing, MI 48824–1117. Email: Schmitt@msu.edu

and now are disappointingly low. This fact is alluded to in the article by Judge (this issue). Barrick and Mount (1991) had available nearly the same set of validity studies when they did their meta-analysis as did Guion and Gottier and both concluded that observed validities did not often exceed .10. Using corrections for unreliability in both predictor and criterion and range restriction, Barrick and Mount estimated that the population validity of conscientiousness was in the mid teens (or mid 20s for subjective criteria). The ensuing rush to use personality in selection that has occurred over the last decade or so since the Barrick and Mount review has been as unthinking, uncritical, and perhaps misguided as was the earlier response to Guion and Gottier (1965). The observed validity of personality measures, then and now, is quite low even though they can account for incrementally useful levels of variance in work-related criteria beyond that afforded by cognitive ability measures because personality and cognitive ability measures are usually minimally correlated.

Likewise, some have expressed reservations about the universality of the Big Five constructs (e.g., Hough, 1998), but they have been accepted by most researchers as representative of the domain of personality. The three articles in this volume represent thoughtful extensions of personality research that challenge both of the accepted "truths" described earlier in at least two respects. First, they go beyond the Big Five to present the development and evaluation of measures of new constructs that may be correlated with some dimensions of the Big Five, but appear not to be simple alternate measures of these dimensions. Secondly, all three articles demonstrate that with careful conceptualization and scale development work, the relatively low observed validities that were observed by both Guion and Gottier (1965) and Barrick and Mount (1991) can be significantly improved.

Two of the articles are strikingly similar in that they approach personality in very cognitive terms. The James, McIntyre, Glisson, Bowler, and Mitchell (this issue) effort focuses on the justification or reasoning behind courses of action to develop a measure of aggression. James (1998) previously espoused this conditional reasoning (CR) approach to the development of measures of other personality constructs as well. Chan (this issue) analyzes two systems of logic—one in which reality is framed in terms of two mutually exclusive categories (e.g., good or evil) and another, based on fuzzy logic, in which the world is perceived in shades of gray or relative levels of ambiguity or goodness and badness. Based on these analyses, Chan develops an individual difference measure of the tolerance for contradiction and tests several hypotheses about relations between this measure and other individual difference measures. These very cognitive approaches to the conceptualization of personality contrast sharply with emotional or affect-laden conceptualizations (George, 1996; Larson, Diener, & Lucas, 2002). The core self-evaluation (CSE) concept and measure described by Judge (this issue) includes cognitive components (e.g., one's view of control and beliefs about self-efficacy), but is also affect laden (e.g., feelings of hopelessness and depression).

Aside from the fact that it is intellectually interesting, this focus on the cognitive nature of individual differences in personality may be important for three reasons. First, I suspect that the more cognitive measures would be less susceptible to coaching, demand characteristics, or attempts at self-aggrandizement. Second, and this may not be a positive feature, it seems to me that they would be related to cognitive ability or verbal comprehension, if for no other reason than that items in both these measures almost have to be verbally complex. Both Chan (this issue) and James et al. (this issue) present information that indicates low or near zero correlations with cognitive ability, but their samples may not have been heterogeneous enough to allow for much variability on the cognitive dimension. Earlier work (James, 1998) on a CR test of achievement motivation indicates a substantial correlation with critical intellectual skills as measured by the American College Testing service. Third, the relatively cognitive nature of these measures means that they are likely more distinct from the typical affect-laden personality measure. This seems to be true as correlations with Chan's measure and Big Five measures ranged from –.19 to .06. James et al. do not present correlations with the Big Five per se, but correlations with other self-report measures suggest that the correlations would be low. Similar correlations for Judge's (this issue) CSE measure are relatively high and, as I suggest later, may indicate that Judge's measure is not empirically distinct from Big Five measures. Given these general observations, the following represents commentary on each of the individual articles and a summary of what I believe we can learn of a general nature from these three articles.

CHAN'S MEASURE OF TOLERANCE FOR CONTRADICTION

The first important thing to note about the measure presented by Chan is that its correlation with performance is near zero. Its utility derives from the fact that it moderates the relation between situational judgment and performance. The obvious next question assuming this relatively large moderator effect is replicated is the extent to which tolerance for contradiction will moderate other predictor–criterion relations. Chan presents good theoretical arguments to predict that the situational judgment and performance relation will be moderated in this fashion, but can these arguments be extended to other predictors and will there be empirical verifications of such moderator effects? Certainly this question should lead to additional research. Chan mentions that the type of outcome measure assessed will affect the degree of the impact of tolerance for contradiction, which is very likely true, but it is really the predictor–criterion relation that needs to be the focus of theory and research. Such theorizing will require more careful thought than the development of rationale for the investigation of the usual bivariate relations (i.e., predictor and criterion). In this context, it will be useful to theorize and test the degree to which the tolerance for contradiction measure is directly related to aspects of performance in some job situations. For example, some have theorized that a tolerance for ambiguity is important in managerial jobs.

Because prediction of performance in this instance is enhanced by an interaction, a practical question relates to whether and how this information might be used to select applicants for a job. What this interaction means is that those low on tolerance for contradiction would be penalized in a selection context if they received high scores on a situational judgment measure. This would be very difficult to justify to applicants or others who might be trying to understand the rationale for selection decisions. This does not, of course, detract from the scientific value or understanding of human performance provided by the results reported in this article, but it may limit the acceptance of this measure in applied contexts.

Chan (this issue) also recognizes the possibility of job by tolerance for contradiction by situational judgment interactions. These interactions seem particularly likely. In the case of the prison guards studied by Chan, it seems to me that if you have no situational judgment capability, you will need to be rigid with respect to following the rules to perform your job adequately and safely. If you have good judgment, it might be the case that a less rigid application of policy would enhance performance. In a different job, in which following procedural guides may not be so critical, a tolerance for contradiction may not have the same impact on the relation between situational judgment and performance.

There were some other, less important considerations with the Chan research. Chan's outline of expected relations with other variables is excellent and for the most part his expectations are supported and do provide evidence for the construct validity of his measure. The small, but significant negative correlation, with Conscientiousness was not expected. Post hoc, I think this relation may be conceptually reasonable. One could expect that those high on Conscientiousness would have relatively low levels of tolerance for contradictions. Chan states that individuals who are high on Conscientiousness are "organized, systematic, and purposeful," characteristics that seem inconsistent with a tolerance for contradictions.

Quite correctly, Chan provides a test for invariance across study participants in his two studies. The test for error variances revealed a significant difference that is not considered meaningful insofar as indicating any measurement differences between college students and prison officers. Judging from the range of trait factor loadings presented for both groups, it appears to be the case that the error variances for the prison officer group were larger. The confirmatory factor analysis in the Judge (this issue) article for his employed sample yielded similar results in that the hypothesized model did not fit well. In both instances, it appears that the trait factor loadings were smaller and the error variances larger in the nonstudent working sample. This may be a simple coincidence, but it may also be worthy of more serious thought and research. Is it possible that students do not distinguish the content in items thought to measure a single construct as clearly as do workers for whom the items may be more meaningful. Or, are the working samples not as careful in responding to the items and more often fail to notice construct similarities? Error variances and corresponding trait factor loadings are quite different in Chan's prison sample and his student sample; if this is true in other studies comparing working and nonworking research participants, it may bear future attention.

Although the exposition of the nomological net considered in collecting evidence about the tolerance for contradictions is excellent, there is one set of constructs that might be considered in future work. Issues of justice come to mind immediately in the context of a tolerance for ambiguity. A major component of the issues considered to be relevant to procedural justice in making decisions about people (e.g., hiring, performance appraisal, salary recommendations) involves items that reduce ambiguity in the manner in which decisions are made. It seems that someone who has a low tolerance for contradictions would be especially sensitive to procedures that cannot be explained by reference to some set of rules. So I would hypothesize that those who cannot tolerate contradictions would be especially sensitive to violations of what they consider procedural justice.

Tolerance for contradictions seems to present us with an interesting and novel individual difference construct that has the potential to explain important work behaviors. Whether it can be used as a decision aid in selection or to make other human resource decisions remains to be demonstrated. Its interaction with situational judgment in this research adds to prediction of job performance at a useful level, but its use may generate objections from those affected by the decisions.

JUDGE'S CSE

Whereas Chan (this issue) and James et al. (this issue) narrow the focus on a specific novel aspect of personality, Judge et al. (this issue) combines measures of four constructs or traits (locus of control, self-esteem, generalized self-efficacy, and emotional stability [neuroticism in its negative version]) into what he has termed CSE. One of Judge's arguments is that measures of these four traits, previously considered separately in the psychological literature, are indicators of a general CSE construct. Over several years and several studies, Judge has built a case for the importance of the CSE construct in work and life satisfaction and job performance. In the article presented in this issue, Judge et al. again report relatively high correlations between a new measure of this general construct and several self-report outcomes. Judge et al.'s arguments about the importance of generalized affect seem convincing and are consistent with a large body of research in many domains (Diener, Suh, Lucas, & Smith, 1999). However, some evidence about the combination of traits espoused by Judge remains ambiguous.

Before we examine this evidence, however, I think it is important to point out that Judge et al.'s work is the first of which I am aware that attempts to explain why personality measures or constructs are related to job performance. Information as to what sorts of motivational sets are the result of given aspects of personality and how these lead to different levels of performance could well lead to better understanding and more effective interventions to increase performance and worker satisfaction. The finding reported in two previous studies that CSE influences job satisfaction in part because more positive individuals obtain more challenging jobs and because they perceive equally complex jobs as more challenging is quite interesting. Highly positive persons appear to get themselves into better situations and perceive the same situations more favorably than less positive persons. We should see that CSE relates to a variety of desirable personal outcomes and one can speculate that CSE will have a cumulative effect over a lifetime. In fact, the long-term and pervasive effects of a positive personality have been investigated by others (Diener & Seligman, 2002; Lucas & Diener, 2003; Staw, Bell, & Clausen, 1986). These other research programs should also be related to Judge's work.

There are some inconsistencies in the argument that locus of control, emotional stability, self-esteem, and generalized self-efficacy are all aspects of CSE and the argument that CSE differs from the Big Five constructs, in particular, Neuroticism. Judge et al. (this issue), in fact, seem to be ambiguous as to whether CSE ought to be considered an alternate operationalization of Emotional Stability. In examining convergent validity and the data presented in Table 1, the argument is that all four constituent traits (at least as measured here) are measures of the same construct. These correlations are all corrected for unreliability so we are talking about the relations between the underlying constructs represented by these measures and the upper limit of the correlations should be 1.00. Only the correlation between self-esteem and generalized self-efficacy approaches 1.00 (i.e., .85). The correlations of locus of control, especially, are notably moderate (average of .53). In Table 2, used as a demonstration that CSE has discriminant validity relative to measures of the Big Five, we see that the correlations of self-esteem, generalized self-efficacy, and locus of control with Neuroticism average −.59. Correlations (absolute values) of all four core measures with Extraversion average .40 and with Conscientiousness, the average is .47. So roughly the same correlations that are taken as evidence of convergence in one table are considered evidence of discriminant validity in the next table. In fairness, Judge et al. take these correlations with Conscientiousness and extraversion as evidence that CSE is a broader concept indicated by a composite of three Big Five traits. It remains the case, however, that in one case, the divergent correlations are actually higher than the convergent correlations. Based on these data, I would question the conclusion that all four of these traits are measures of the same general construct. Especially in the case of locus of control, these data were not convincing.

Even the correlation (corrected for unreliability in both measures) between the new measure of CSE and Neuroticism is −.81 (uncorrected r in Table 4 is −.66). Here this correlation is presented as evidence that "emotional stability does not represent this broad construct" (i.e., CSE). This correlation is nearly as large as the largest of the correlations in Table 1, all of which are presented as evidence that the four core traits are aspects of the *same* construct. Divergence and convergence appear to be very much in the eye of the beholder and the beholder is not consistent!

In the interest of parsimony, it is certainly laudable that Judge et al. and the other authors in this special issue provide correlations between their new measures and the Big Five. In the case of this article, though, I wondered why measures of positive and negative affect (Watson, Clark, & Tellegen, 1988) or measures from the Diener and Seligman (2002) or Staw et al. (1986) work were not included. Certainly, the conceptual basis for examining the correlation with measures of affect was available in the article; empirical estimation of the correlations seems like an obvious requirement in this research program. It is the case that measures of positive and negative affect do not include the control aspect that is conceptually part of CSE but, as mentioned earlier, I am questioning the appropriateness of its inclusion in the CSE construct.

Judge et al. also argued that the relatively broad CSE measure should predict broad criteria better than measures of the four individual traits that go into the CSE concept. They cite data from two studies that indicate CSE predicts job performance, motivation, and life and job satisfaction better than any single measure of the four traits. This is undoubtedly the case if the individual traits are correlated with an outcome and with each other. Arithmetically, this has to be the case. What would be more supportive of CSE would be evidence that this new measure of CSE has superior validity to a composite of the four measures. If this is the case, or the much shorter measure of CSE presented in this article has validity superior to that afforded by a composite of the four individual traits, then we have something new and a potentially more parsimonious explanation of behavior. Based on the evidence presented in this article, I doubt that would be the case.

Table 5 of the Judge et al. (this issue) article contains CFA results for three respondent samples. As noted earlier in discussing the results of the Chan work, the CFA for the employee sample yields what appears to be less favorable evidence with respect to the unidimensionality of the CSE measure than is the case for the other two samples. Whether this lack of fit in employed or "real-world" samples is coincidental or the product of reliably different perceptions of work-related constructs may be the focus of future inquiry. I also wonder how the author achieved 50 degrees of freedom in these models. There should be 54 (78 pieces of information with 12 factor loadings and 12 error variances estimated). If estimates of other parameters were necessary to achieve the levels of fit reported in this table, this should be reported and may change conclusions about the unidimensionality of the CSE measure.

In summary, the conceptual arguments for the CSE measure and the need for parsimony of explanation, as well as the practical need for parsimony in the number of measures and items included in our research, all suggest that the CSE measure may represent a real advance in the study of personality. In addition, the exploration of the mediating mechanisms involved in personality–performance relations is overdue and laudable. However, the empirical data supporting the existence of a single CSE construct and its independence from other constructs seem to be more favorably described and interpreted than is warranted.

JAMES ET AL. CR

James et al. (this issue) presents impressive evidence concerning the validity of their measure of aggression using the CR approach just as they have earlier in the case of achievement motivation (James, 1998). This cognitively based approach to personality measurement is certainly a significant departure from the usual personality instrument and it seems that it should be more resistant to deliberate attempts to present oneself favorably. I do have several conceptual comments or questions though and several perhaps less important questions related to the data presented in the James et al. article.

First, based on the first two attempts of James et al. to develop measures based on CR, it seems that the technique is more readily adapted to the measure of traits that have negative social consequences. Particularly in the case of aggression, all the justification mechanisms are negative. It seems to me that there is a positive side to aggression as well. A new faculty member who is not aggressive in seeking the resources to launch a successful program of research and who does not pursue her or his goals with some level of initiative and aggression is destined to fail. In most life situations, it seems that some level of what I interpret to be aggression is necessary if one is to achieve either personal, family, or societal goals. James et al. may take this logic as evidence of the author's tendency to be aggressive versus prosocial, but it seems that James is setting up the CR paradigm to measure undesirable traits. This also seemed to be the case in developing a measure of achievement motivation (see James, 1998). This tendency to view aggression as negative is obvious in the table representing the justification mechanisms as well as the example item that is analyzed. So, the question is whether or not CR can be used to develop measures of "positive" traits, such as extraversion or altruism, or would we have to start with introversion and self-interest and work to build items that justify the avoidance of people and considering only one's self-interest in deciding on a course of behavior? Even when James et al. provide examples of positive behaviors at the end of the article, they frame them as the opposites of a negative trait.

Second, James et al. (this issue) claims that the CR approach is resistant to faking or self- enhancement. If one reads the example items and considers the manner in which items are developed and the relatively indirect ways in which scoring protocols are developed, this certainly seems like a reasonable claim. In reading example items, however, I suspect that if respondents were given minimal instruction on the nature of the targeted construct and asked to respond in a given direction, their scores would change. James has not yet provided empirical evidence of the claims regarding the CR measures resistance to faking and studies of the impact of motivation and coaching on scores on these measures should be high on their and others' research agenda. Correlations with measures of impression management may also be informative.

It is not obvious to me how one generates a CR item, though it seems that much more thought and planning and tryout is required than is the case for the typical Likert-type or checklist items we see in most personality measures. Beyond some very general discussion, there is little guidance in the article in this issue of *Human Performance* or in the earlier article by James (1998) that would allow interested others to develop a CR measure. This is especially critical to any widespread use of the technique to measure other personality dimensions or even to use the measures that are developed. It is both understandable and disappointing that these measures now appear to be copyrighted (James & McIntyre, 2000). Perhaps such a volume or article now exists, but I think it would be helpful if James and his colleagues produced a manual that details how they have developed these measures, especially if access to currently developed measures will be limited.

As mentioned earlier, I had a number of questions about the data presented in this article. I am not sure conceptually why aggression should be related to job performance. In some jobs, like that of a police officer for which James presents one set of validity data, this might be reasonable. That is, a highly aggressive police officer may get himself or herself and a police department in trouble. However, it seems that a more direct test of the job-relatedness of the aggression measure would be to correlate it with the number and severity of disciplinary problems faced by officers rather than any overall measure of performance. James et al. (this issue) present a large number of validity coefficients with other more appropriate criteria and this certainly represents the strongest evidence for the utility of their approach to personality measurement. These coefficients are really quite radically superior to the existing literature on the validity of personality measures.

James et al. (this issue) presents a verbal description of the factor analysis of their aggression measure and report that this factor analysis confirmed the existence of five of the six justification mechanisms that were built into the measure. It would be helpful to know where the items that represented the Derogation of Bias mechanism loaded in this five-factor solution. Likewise, the alphas for the five remaining factors are presented, but their intercorrelations are not. Both are critical if we are to draw any conclusions about the nature of the distinctiveness of these five dimensions. I assume that the authors decided that there was little evidence for dimensionality (see the results regarding the KR–20) because they used a composite measure in the remainder of the analyses discussed. Also, in discussing the reliability of these measures, I do not see why or actually how the authors applied the KR–20 formula to the computation of reliability. This estimate of reliability is appropriate for dichotomously scored items and the James et al. items were scored using a three-point scale (+1, 0, −1). It would be helpful to know how and why the items were dichotomized to produce a KR–20 estimate of reliability.

Several comments made by James et al. regarding personality measures in general are well taken. The factors that were troublesome about personality measurement in the 1960s are still present. As noted at the outset, the low observed validities for personality measures reported by Guion and Gottier (1965) have not disappeared. We have corrected them away. These corrections do provide the relations between constructs, but they also seem to excuse continued use of lousy measures and do not relate to their practical utility (Murphy & DeShon, 1998). The science and practice of personality measurement would be well served by more frequent direct attempts to increase the quality of measurement as opposed to simply correcting away deficiencies on the basis of questionable assumptions.

GENERAL COMMENTS AND SUMMARY

Another general observation about these three programs of research on personality is interesting. None of these authors seems to have started their work with a job analysis or the nature of work on a specific job or occupation—the way industrial/organizational psychologists usually engage in test development and validation work. They started with observations about the nature of personality variables across many situations in which they have been investigated (Judge, this issue), different ways of viewing the world (Chan, this issue), and the nature of the reasoning one applies to the choice of behavioral actions (James et al., this issue). These general observations or theories about human behavior are then applied to the behavior of people at work. All three programs of research provide the basis for considerable optimism about the theoretical and practical utility of the target measures. If we are to generalize to other efforts toward progress in measuring and understanding personality, these experiences suggest that we should draw on organizational science, psychology, and related behavioral science disciplines to better inform theory. As stated earlier, we should also draw on our sophistication in measurement; each of these programs of research involved careful consideration of measurement issues, the collection of a variety of supporting data, and its thorough analysis.

Although all three programs of research provide encouraging results, I am sure that all three sets of authors would agree that much remains to be done. For Chan, it seems that the most important question involves the replication and generalization of his results to other jobs, criteria, and predictor–criterion relations. For James et al., I think it will be most important to provide information to others on how to develop a CR measure, how to extend this research to "positive" constructs, and to provide evidence that these measures are indeed not as susceptible to self-enhancement as traditional personality measures. Finally, for Judge et al., I think it will be most useful if further studies of the degree to which CSE actually measures a novel construct were undertaken. If that seems to be the case, then more investigations of the relations among CSE and other personality measures that appear (to me, at least) to be theoretically similar (e.g., positive affectivity) should be conducted. Finally, it seems that longitudinal research on this construct and how its apparently beneficial implications accumulate across time would be very interesting.

REFERENCES

Barrick, M. R., & Mount, M. K. (1991). The Big Five personality dimensions and job performance: A meta-analysis. *Personnel Psychology, 44*, 1–26.

Costa, P. T., & McRae, R. R. (1988). Personality in adulthood: A six-year longitudinal study of self-reports and spouse ratings on the NEO Personality Inventory. *Journal of Personality and Social Psychology, 54*, 853–863.

Diener, E., & Seligman, M. E. P. (2002). Very happy people. *Psychological Science, 13*, 81–84.

Diener, E., Suh, E. M., Lucas, R. E., & Smith, H. (1999). Subjective well-being: Thirty years of progress. *Psychological Bulletin, 125*, 276–302.

George, J. M. (1996). Trait and state affect. In K. R. Murphy (Ed.), *Individual differences and behavior in organizations* (pp. 145–171). San Francisco: Jossey-Bass.

Guion, R. M., & Gottier, R. F. (1965). Validity of personality measures in personnel selection. *Personnel Psychology, 18*, 135–164.

Hough, L. (1998). Personality at work: Issues and evidence. In M. D. Hakel (Ed.), *Beyond multiple choice: Evaluating alternatives to traditional testing for selection* (pp. 131–166). Mahwah, NJ: Lawrence Erlbaum Associates, Inc.

James, L. R. (1998). Measurement of personality via conditional reasoning. *Organizational Research Methods, 1*, 131–163.

James, L. R., & McIntyre, M. D. (2000). *Conditional Reasoning Test of Aggression test manual*. San Antonio, TX: Psychological Corporation.

Larsen, R. J., Diener, E., & Lucas, R. E. (2002). Emotion: Models, measures, and individual differences. In R. G. Lord, R. J. Klimoski, & R. Kanfer (Eds.), *Emotions in the workplace* (pp. 64–106). San Francisco: Jossey-Bass.

Lucas, R. E., & Diener, E. (2003). The happy worker: Hypotheses about the role of positive affect in worker productivity. In M. R. Barrick & A. M. Ryan (Eds.), *Personality and work: Reconsidering the role of personality in organizations* (pp. 30–59). San Francisco: Jossey-Bass.

Murphy, K. R., & DeShon, R. P. (1998). Progress in psychometrics: Can industrial and organizational psychology catch up? *Personnel Psychology, 53*, 913–924.

Staw, B. M., Bell, N. E., & Clausen, J. A. (1986). The dispositional approach to job attitudes: A lifetime longitudinal test. *Administrative Science Quarterly, 31*, 56–77.

Watson, D., Clark, L. A., & Tellegen, A. (1988). Development and validation of brief measures of positive and negative affect: The PANAS Scales. *Journal of Personality and Social Psychology, 54*, 1063–1070.

Instructions for Authors

Human Performance publishes research on the nature of performance in the workplace and in applied settings, and encourages submission of papers that go beyond the study of traditional job behavior.

Submissions to *Human Performance* will be evaluated according to several different criteria: significance, adequacy of design and of execution of study, integrity of analyses, quality of introduction and discussion, clarity of expression, and extent to which the manuscript addresses the emphasis of the journal. Under certain circumstances, we will accept replications and studies in which the null hypothesis is not rejected; these circumstances are described in the Editorial Statement that appears in Volume 1, Number 1. The following instructions for authors have been developed from and follow closely the guidelines adopted and published by journals of the American Psychological Association (APA).

Manuscripts should conform to the guidelines presented in the *Publication Manual of the American Psychological Association* (5th ed., 2001); manuscripts that do not adhere to these guidelines will be returned without being reviewed. Manuscripts should include a 100- to 150-word abstract typed on a separate sheet of paper. All text (including tables, footnotes, and references) should be double-spaced, and all sexist language should be eliminated. There is no limit on length: Manuscripts can vary from short notes of 6 to 10 manuscript pages to monographs of 70 pages or more.

We will follow the APA policy that authors not submit a manuscript to more than one source at the same time. Authors should state in a cover letter that the manuscript is not under consideration for publication elsewhere; similarly, we will not accept a manuscript that has appeared (or that will appear) in any other source in whole or substantial part. Authors should also state in the cover letter that they have followed the APA ethical standards for the treatment of human or animal subjects. These guidelines are available from the American Psychological Association Ethics Office, 750 First Street, NE, Washington, DC 20002–4242.

Four copies of each manuscript should be submitted for publication consideration. Unless otherwise requested, reviews will not be anonymous. When anonymous reviews are requested, the name and affiliation of the author, as well as any other identifying information, should not appear in the body of the manuscript or author notes. A separate title page should appear on each copy of a manuscript for which an anonymous review is requested.

Manuscripts should be mailed to the Editor, James L. Farr, Ph.D., *Human Performance,* Department of Psychology, 615 Moore Building, The Pennsylvania State University, University Park, PA 16802–3104.